The **Way** of
Arnold

Experiencing Your Full Potential
While Turning Back the Clock
With Every Loving Raw Moment

ARNOLD N. KAUFFMAN
Owner of Arnold's Way

Copyright and Other Information

Medical and Exercise Disclaimers

This book is not intended as a substitute for the medical advice of physicians. The reader should regularly consult a physician in matters relating to his or her health and particularly with respect to any symptoms that may require diagnosis or medical attention. The opinions expressed in this book are made by the author only, and the reader takes full responsibility for taking and using the advice provided herein.

The information in this book is meant to supplement, not replace, proper rebounder training. Like any sport involving speed, equipment, balance and environmental factors, rebounding poses some inherent risk. The author and publisher advise readers to take full responsibility for their safety and know their limits. Before practicing the skills described in this book, be sure your equipment is well-maintained. Do not take risks beyond your level of experience, aptitude, training and comfort level.

<u>Acknowledgments</u>

There are many individuals who have shaped my raw foods fruitarian journey. I would like to take this space to acknowledge their contributions to my effort:

Brian Rossiter (Fruit-Powered.com), without whose help, this book would never be done. He took this book from the depths of nothingness to its full fruition. He works countless hours not only helping me, but more important, spreading the word of raw potential and how it can affect every human being. They can be free of disease, depression, anxiety and have continuous hope that their lives can be lived to their full potential. On that note, I give great thanks to Brian.

Joy King, who took my spoken words and scribbled writing and dedicated herself to making my dream of writing a book into a reality. She spent countless hours turning my ideas into a legible form.

Sheryl Sankey, who came to me and volunteered her services to edit and unscramble my project of words and thought processes into book form. Her service was not to help me but help free the world of disease. She worked countless hours to turn this dream into reality.

Megan Elizabeth (MeganElizabeth.com), who worked with me for three-and-a-half years. She called me her mentor, and she became one of my heroes. Her existence reeks of purity and excellence, and she finished her book, inspiring me to write mine as a service of what to do and what not to do. I thank her greatly.

Stephanie Greene, who continually encouraged me to write my book and stepped in when no one was available to help finish typing the book.

About the Author

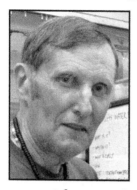

Arnold Kauffman, 65, consumes mostly fruits and greens and always says he is getting younger every day! As quoted on YouTube.com, "Arnold's body is a specimen of what the male body should look like!"

Arnold has owned Arnold's Way Vegetarian Raw Café and Health Center since 1992. After starting as a vitamin store, Arnold's Way evolved, beginning to focus on Natural Hygiene and a fruitarian-based raw foods lifestyle for exceptional health in 1998. Located outside Philadelphia, the Lansdale, Pennsylvania, café is a worldwide destination for young and old exploring and leading raw foods lifestyles. Arnold has educated thousands to eat raw foods and many to transition to mostly or wholly raw lifestyles. He's also taught many how they can reverse health challenges by creating optimum healing conditions for their bodies.

Arnold works 75 to 100 hours a week on his mission: "To create an energetic movement for the transformation to a disease-free world!" He offers classes and workshops and hands out free samples of green smoothies and banana whips at community events.

Arnold has been featured on the Fox affiliate and PBS member station in Philadelphia and has been written about in several publications, including *The Philadelphia Inquirer*, *The Reporter* (Lansdale, Pennsylvania) and *Vibrance*.

Table of Contents

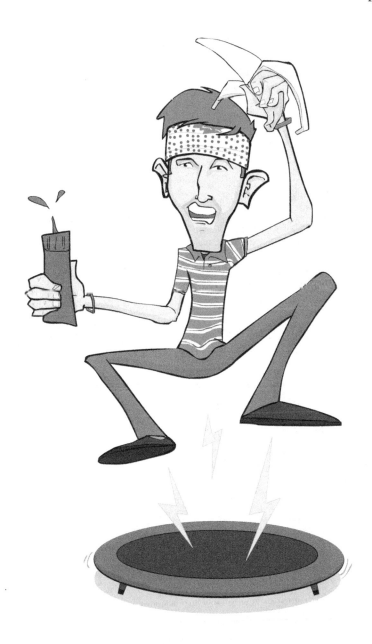

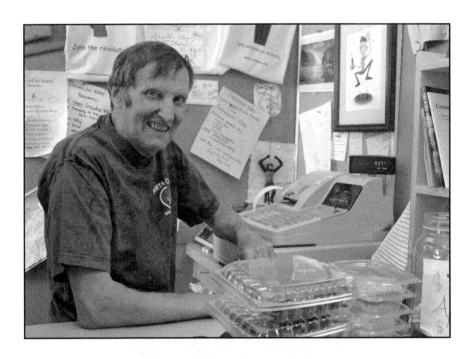

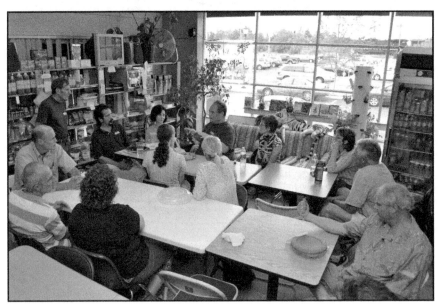

Introduction

WE BREATHE, WORK AND THINK. We live by the way we were raised.

These thoughts, attitudes and lifestyle choices reflect how I think, as of today.

As of today and as of yesterday, we are in a continual state of flow that is our reality, and I mean *our reality*. I give thanks for the future and am in a continual state of gratitude.

As I write my words, I think of the diseases that ravish my town, country and world. I think of the harmonic flow that nature is so desperately seeking to manifest, and I do mean desperately not just to maintain but to survive against man and woman's barrages of chemical warfare. As the world is total and complete, so is our body singularly complete. Our bodies are a microcosm of the world that exists outside ourselves. Our bodies can feel like a troubling and poisonous overflow of rivers and streams that is destroying our internal mechanism, not only for ourselves, but for each succeeding generation. If we don't honor them with the right dietary choices, our health will begin a slow degeneration. This book is dedicated to preventing that from happening. Our bodies should act like a harmonic rhapsody, blue symmetry that purrs with pure delight.

Our bodies want to flow in accordance with harmony and love. Our 75 trillion cells work in unison to create a state of utter perfection. It's the 20,000 units in each individual cell that create the magnificent force of mechanisms. The magnificence of the body is more luminous than all the brilliance that ever existed in our modern world put together. The body and mind have an innate intelligence that works so efficiently and magnificently that we are oblivious to the way each organ, each tissue and each part of our bodies functions automatically. Still, my life continues knowing this energetic vibration of truth and without abiding by the code of every food choice.

My overriding philosophy, in my opinion, is that we need not be authentically pure, especially on a moment-by-moment basis. The key is to add more fruits and greens in your dietary practice. The body's wisdom will then do the rest.

I am continually enamored about how our bodies are engrossed in a multitude of activities, working endlessly to create continual purification and homeostasis. It is mind-boggling that all these zillions of activities are going on inside us just to create a moment of life.

This book is dedicated to those readers who desire to live by rules that stem from a higher place—a place that deals with truth, honesty and harmony. To me, there are no shades of gray. I think they are nonexistent because they simply don't work in a body that thrives on excellence. The rules that determine our existence—such as how our heart beats, what we see, what we hear, what we understand and how all this is interpreted—also play an integral role in how we deal with truth in life.

I dedicate this book to not only my well-being but to that of my readers because I have no choice in the matter. I believe it is my job to share with others the truth of what I believe and what I understand.

We live in a world where the way to peace and harmony (which is found within, supposedly) is constantly being bombarded by mass media propaganda. We are inundated with so much factual information being presented by so-called authoritarian representatives. It is almost impossible to gain a clear understanding of our truth, which has its own built-in wisdom on how life should be lived.

I take my understanding, my 20 years of experience in dealing with physical and emotional disease and state out loud and clear that most of these diseases are self-created and that we have the ability to undo what does not have to be. It is with this understanding that I am driven not only to write this book but to use my life force, will and passion as a guide post for others to be able to say, "I am responsible for my health."

As the owner of Arnold's Way, a raw vegan café, health food store and educational meeting space in Lansdale, Pennsylvania, I hear, read and deal with basically every known disease. Every day I see, read and hear people dying of cancer, diabetes and other diseases. I see children and adults who are overweight, and I get questioned all the time: "Well, what do you do?"

This book is dedicated to all those people who want to change their lives by taking charge of their health and eliminating dependency on the health-care field. This book is not only about me, it's about how I started Arnold's Way.

I will share with you how I started Arnold's Way and what drives me almost to the point of total obsession seven days a week, 10 to 12 hours a day. I live with the understanding that what I do is because of my drive, passion and desire to be in total harmony not only with those around me but, more important, to be in flow with myself. More important, I want to share that understanding with others to help them find their path in finding their own truth.

How I came to choose the raw lifestyle as my purpose for living came into being by my sense of seeking truth in my daily existence. We live in a kind of tangible world where seconds really do matter. This realization is so incredible that if I would have had 10 consecutive sneezes, I would have missed my whole direction, path and, literally, my reason for being here and who I am today. I would not be in excellent health, an inspiration to thousands of others, and, most likely, I would be just another average 65-year-old man using sayings like, "Hang in there," "I'm surviving," "What's up with the coffee machine?" and "Who's winning?" All these thoughts that could have been came swishing into my head.

I often wonder if I would have even made it to that age. I probably would have had a lot of aches and pains, be collecting Social Security and reconciling myself to the feeling that the best years of my life have passed me by with each passing day. I would have been very slowly stepping into a world of slow decline had I had not moved forward and upward in accordance with my primary inner voice for what I should be and do the rest of life. This overriding desire for peace and harmony motivated me to embark on a journey that has enabled me to experience unbelievable health and ecstatic well-being on a moment-to-moment basis.

I can say more about the turns my life could have taken, but I think it is more helpful to share with you a few fun-filled, exciting and exhilarating circumstances that turned my life around in an amazing way.

Chapter 1

A Visit from the Angels Above

IT WAS ONE OF THOSE SUNNY August days that wasn't really different from any other day. I was a young man of 25 years who thought I knew how to court pretty women. I continually chased them till I caught them and then quickly tossed them aside like rotted fish that remained too long in the refrigerator. At the time and, still, even today, I would run away, fearful, carried away by my youthful innocence and afraid that I'd be forever trapped in a box in gray and black shreds of worn-out duct tape if I ever did so get involved in a romantic relationship.

So I filled myself with bottles of beer, going to bars, and looking for something to do because that was the thing to do, with a drink-till-ya-get-drunk attitude. Back then, I was no different from anyone else. I wanted to experience the taste of freedom! These were my days of summer 1972. I was single, free and full of hope. I also had a clear understanding that life was already planned for me by the powers to be. I barely knew that I was even in that game of being molded, like a tiny pattern figure being cut and sized. Nevertheless, I was in that mindset that I would go to college, get a job for 30 years, get married, buy a house, have and raise kids. It all so seemed so controlled, with all the borders well-defined. And it all seemed so harmless. At the time, this lifestyle approach seemed as if it were the only way to live, think and be.

At the time, I felt obligated to live the American dream—doing anything else was not the norm.

If truth be truth, all these things did happen. This is how my life unfolded. This is how I lived. I got married, raised kids and thought, "This is the way people should live their lives." I thought this was how it was all going to play out till the very end of my existence—in fact all this would've happened except for this one tiny blip of a moment in time back then when I felt I received a whack from a hard baseball bat that buzzed and barely missed my helmet. It was like a *kahbang*, like a lightning bolt that had my name on it.

Call it damn crazy, weird and totally off the wall, but I felt as if I was touched by a higher power right in the middle of the street. I felt as if this higher power was whispering into my ear, "Arnold, go forth in this world and be the light so others can see." My friends, *this* became my calling. *This* became the start of my life passion, my every reason for doing what I do now. And now my socks are completely knocked off. Being here for others is the love of my life. It is such a gift. What a blessing!

It is my belief that we, as a people, all have that same calling. My moment in change happened when I was standing right in the middle of the street at 13th and Pine streets in Philadelphia, innocently crossing over from the old Not Just Ice Cream parlor, where I had just eaten the most delicious ice cream, and heading over to the corner pizza shop for a slice of pizza with mushrooms. I felt as if I was tapped on the shoulder by an angelic presence. I was totally aghast, totally mesmerized and totally in danger because I couldn't move. I was too afraid and in a state of pure shock. I didn't want to miss a single word that was being delivered to me by a divine presence.

Somehow I sensed I was having a life-altering experience at that moment in time. I also knew I could not fathom the magnitude of words spoken to me. It was about 40 years ago that I stood dazed, listening to the words that struck me right there in the middle of the street, where I was too stunned to move. I looked around to see if anybody saw anything. There was no one in sight. I took the words and held them deeply within my inner being. I took this revelation and just tucked it away and buried it deep within the recesses of my mind for at the time it was simply not *the* time. At the time, I was a simple man living a simple life, doing the best I could as I am now, 40 years later.

The words became a memory to cherish, to hold dear to my heart and to abide within me until they could be reignited when the moment was right. At the time, I was a flaming arrow, full of ambition, life and thoughts. I didn't think so much about me but about world peace, world harmony, world complexity and about how everything is so real and yet so fragile. It was more than I could figure out then as well as today. At the time, I was looking for solutions. I sought out an answer and couldn't think of a way to live in harmony any longer in the United States, so I decided to move to Israel. I knew what I wanted: the peace, harmony and passion I could no longer find while living in the United States.

Israel, I believed at the time, was my home and ancestry. It embodied my vision as a new and fresh start in life. It was the case then as it is now that part of my journey and part of my destiny is to seek the peace and harmony that each of us so truly desires. I wanted to get up with the rising of the sun, hear the cackling of the birds and feel the dew on the grass surrounding me and move in that harmonic flow of life every moment of my life.

I thought of Israel as my final destination. It was to be my home of homes. At the time, my every thought and every action was to leave the United States for good to go live in Israel. During the next 20 years, I traveled to Israel, left Israel, got married and had kids. Without my family and kids, all this would be for naught. In my deepest thoughts and emotions, I know having a family is the most worthwhile thing. Otherwise, nothing really matters. I want to give humble thanks to my ex-wife and children for giving me the true meaning of life.

This first transformative experience when I heard that inner voice directive put me into this omnipresent flow of excitement and exhilaration.

We are always given the opportunity to make choices at any given moment. I write these words to be a beacon of hope and support and a light for others. There is a guiding light in each and every one of us. We have to see, feel and, most important, follow our true passion of being the light within as well as on the outside.

Chapter 2

Let Me Close
Your Eyes Forever

MY SECOND MAJOR TRANSFORMATION happened almost 20 years later, in the summer of 1989. It was also one of those rare occurrences that, had I blinked longer than 10 seconds, I would not be writing these words. It was one of those incidences when it felt as if a lightning bolt struck me so vividly and so fast, that to this day, 23 years later, I am still burning with hot passion caused by that moment.

This transformational change started out as an unintentional possibility without a hint of a provocation. In fact, if anything, it could have been labeled "No big deal." At the time, my then-wife worked at a summer camp where volunteers were hired to work for the season. It was our family's tradition to open our home to any volunteer who needed a place to stay after camp hours. Each year was different, and each year was fun. Each year the family looked forward to having one of the volunteers stay with us.

In 1989, Lucy, a volunteer at the camp, came to stay with us. Lucy was a 22-year-old beautiful artesian, full of life, full of questions, full of insights about herself and the world around her. She talked about the good, the bad and the ugly. On one particular afternoon, Lucy and I happened to be talking in my bright yellow kitchen. It was one of those conversations where gibberish was flowing back and forth. It was a sleepy afternoon in which I was one yawn away from falling asleep. All of a sudden, the conversation took a turn that changed my life and changed my way of thinking forever. Basically, Lucy asked me life altering questions such as "What do I really want?", "What is my calling?", "Am I really happy?" and, finally, "What would it take for me to be happy—truthfully happy?"

Her questions were like sharp daggers striking the essence of my being and permeated every inch of my existence. I realized I was still living an incomplete life. I realized I was not leading the life I was supposed to be living. I had four beautiful children and a lovely wife, lived in a fancy house and held a secure job that was mine until the day I retired. It appeared as if I had the perfect life. But I knew deep inside that I was not happy with my life. A sense of purpose in my life was missing, and at the time, I had no idea what it was.

Lucy's questions were brief, to the point and totally absorbed my thinking. It took me almost six years to have a complete understanding of what these questions meant and how to live the rest of my life based on them. This book, on some level, is a dedication to Lucy.

As the conversation became more intense and I became more absorbed in our communication, Lucy changed her thought process suddenly and handed me a note that said, "Let me close your eyes forever." I recall looking at the words and at her, saying, "What the heck does that mean?" She smiled and before she could explain the meaning of her words, my family began rushing into our home. We never spoke again about that note. The next morning, she drew a picture of a man in a dream state who was at peace with himself. I became inspired to write my first poem in 16 years in honor of her words, her picture and, most important, myself. My creative energy, which was bottled up for all those years, just burst wide open. I became obsessed, for whatever reason, with writing poetry because I was living a life and daily routine that wasn't truly mine for too long.

Thank goodness.

I then became obsessed with discovering what Lucy's words meant. It was as if nothing else mattered. Her words and picture haunted me for years. Day and night, I dived deeply into the recesses of my inner being. My heart was empty, like a big bucket of water that had to be constantly filled because it had a hole in it. There was a deep ache and pain that I had no idea how to fill.

It was not only her words but her note, written in the briefest of words, which, to this day, are deeply embedded in my heart and actions. They are my guiding light, continually creating a life of passion within me. I sit quietly in my rocking chair, looking at my garden, listening to the birds chirp, seeing all of the green that ebbs and flows before my eyes as I think about the conversation we had with each other that fateful day. This conversation changed the course of my life and started me on the road where I am today.

After six months of tortuous analytical observation as to what those words meant, I came across shiatsu. It was the fruition of trying to discover what Lucy's words meant to me. I saw an advertisement in a newspaper on healing through acupressure, and this resonated with me on what was my destination of life's goals and possibilities.

Shiatsu is a Chinese form of healing and acupressure massage. I loved it and connected with it on a very deep level. This form of healing is about touch, love, healing and connecting with others in a space where words are not needed. It was a modality where I could make connections that were about peace and harmony and about being in a sacred place where the total essence of our being is honored. It deals with the real essence of one's soul, and most important, it allows our vulnerability to be our strength. I discovered that touch can be a loving communication form and way to share our true love and nature.

It is my nature to be passionately in love with whatever I do at the moment. At that moment in time, shiatsu resonated with me. As important as my shiatsu discovery was for me, it didn't reflect the total insight of "Let me close your eyes forever." In my heart and soul, I knew there had to be something more. My every thought and action was geared to being at peace with myself. I wanted to feel and be more complete within my mind, body and soul. I wanted to be less angry, less volatile in my temper swings and more loving, not only to my wife and kids, but to myself as well. I started to wake up and realize I deserve to have what I want and be who I want to be and become. At the time, I was afraid of almost everything. I had almost zero self-esteem. I was afraid to open my mouth in any conversation involving more than three people. not to mention that I was deathly afraid of speaking in front of an audience and giving a presentation or talking.

All this is part of the journey, and back then, it became my quest to find out the true essence of those words, "Let me close your eyes forever." I had to discover what they meant for my life and how they would affect the lives of those around me.

Chapter 3

Daily News Headline
Changes My Life

MY THIRD TRANSFORMATIVE CHANGE happened about two years later when I was working at a post office. At that time, I was already deep into shiatsu, studying, learning and diagnosing as an integral part of my being. I then quit working for the Postal Service after 10 years and started a junk-food vending business. I no longer wanted to be part of the bureaucratic system. Both changes were part of my journey.

There is a progression in life. The more we get in tune with finding our purpose in life, the more, I believe, we learn about the purpose of our journey and what our destiny is. Through a series of experiences I will share with you shortly, I became aware that the body is a magnificent life-support system.

There are millions of intricate processes that work together in unison to support and protect the life of the body. I became aware of the subtle and not so-subtle signals the body gives us to let us know that its balance is being thrown off course and that its health or survival is at risk. The body loves us so much that it talks to us moment by moment, letting us know what it needs to support and maintain its optimum health. The body asks only that its primary needs are met such as a species-specific diet, fresh air, clean water, exercise and to love ourselves unconditionally. Our bodies require that we respect its needs and wants. If we are willing to love our bodies as a mother would her newborn baby, our bodies will lovingly respond to our care and attention, and the result will be exquisite health.

These were the kind of thoughts that filled my head. I had no idea where I was supposed to be or go or what I was supposed to do but was open to be in the flow of where life was taking me. I knew I wanted to follow my passion, seek the highest good and listen very intently to what my inner voice had to say about what I want and to determine how badly I wanted to do it.

I was married with four kids. There was always something else to buy and somewhere else to go, and no matter how much money we made, it never seemed to be enough. I got caught up in the material world and wanted to get out. I wanted to change my consciousness about this life I was living at the time. I wanted a change. I kept thinking as an adult: "What was I going to do when I grew up?"

Even though I owned a successful vending machine business, it was not enough. Everything I'm mentioning here was good. I thought I was healthy as well as can be expected for a 44-year-old guy. I was not overweight, weighing about 165 pounds and bearing a 34-inch waist. I was showing some gray hair, and I was heavy in the cheeks. All these things were minor details and did not play a role in my day-to-day existence. Essentially, I was a happy camper on the outside, but in the back of my mind, I was secretly driven by my desire to fulfill my life's purpose with passion.

All of these things were working on my mind on a continual basis as I left a gym and headed to Wendy's for my weekly treat of a cheeseburger with pickles, an order of french fries and a Coke—and, of course, my copy of the *Philadelphia Daily News*.

As I had done before so many times before with the same meal, I found the perfect seat so I could sit down and read in peace and eat my food. Everything was perfect until that very moment when I reached in and grabbed the *Daily News* out of the box.

It was during that moment in time when my life took a miraculous change. Everything in my life that had meaning to me became like fine wood being changed into sawdust. It was at that dramatic life-changing moment when I saw the words on the front page of the *Daily News* in big, bold black letters that jumped out at me like a mugger in New York City, "The Jews are a threat to this society, and we have to find a solution."

These words were spoken by David Duke, who, at the time, was head of the Ku Klux Klan. As I saw these words, I noted they were on the front page of a major newspaper, and I was astounded. At the time, I was just a deliverer of snacks, a very quiet man who disliked speaking in public and was self-conscious about my abilities to communicate with my wife, let alone in front of a large group of people. I had also lived in Israel for five years and was very much into the Zionist movement. I believed then and still do today that Israel should be the home for all Jews. It was somewhere in between these three thoughts that this headline, for whatever reason, came flying at me, grabbed me by the gonads and said, "ARNOLD, DO SOMETHING!"

In that moment, all that I perceived as good, including the foods that lustfully sustained me, came to an abrupt ending. I knew in my heart and soul that if ever there was going to be peace and coexistence between the Jews and Arabs and/or people of all nationalities that I should be equally passionate in helping people find their light as a way to end all wars, hatred and anger.

As it was then and as it is now, I felt that I had to do something. I felt that I had no choice in the matter. Everything I thought was important at the time became a secondary consideration. I, Arnold N. Kauffman, in fall 1991, had suddenly found my purpose and passion all rolled into one. I became driven. I was going to stop this evil destructive thought process that was not only a threat to Jews but to all of mankind. As I understood Duke, it seemed as if he thought that anybody who was a little different—whether in religious belief, color, thought process, sexual orientation or anybody who did not follow the status quo—wasn't considered a true American. These individuals and groups who didn't align themselves with his narrow definition of what it means to be American were considered a threat to the American way of life.

Chapter 4

I Have to Do Something

QUESTIONS REMAINED: "What do I do to stop this maniacal visionary whose idealism was a threat to me? How do I respond to this warped evil sense of purpose and logic that could potentially be the second coming of Nazism in the United States?" In that moment, I literally gave myself permission to do something to create an energetic movement to transform that negative thought process. I saw his thought process as a threat to Israel and me and flawed logic as a vision of Nazism reviving in the United States. That moment, as I was eating that Wendy's meal, became my transforming moment. It was from that moment onward that my life took a dramatic turn.

I was driven to come up with a solution and a doable, nonconfrontational plan that would not only stop this maddening, destructive nonharmonic thought process but transform the world into a place where we could all exist peacefully as it is in nature, where no footprint is left behind. I knew that I needed to make a stand and that I had to discover what my dream, destiny and life's purpose was. I needed to find a vehicle in which I could express this newfound ideal of living my dream, fulfilling my purpose and being true to myself, as God intended.

I thought to myself that if I could change the way people ate, I could change the way they think. I instinctively thought

I had a drive for a calling, and this made it much more clear on what I had to do. I thought that the best way to begin this process of changing the negative attitude of racism was to help people to find alternative solutions to their health concerns by opening a health food store in an area that was open to my way of thinking. I thought that Philadelphia would be the best place to open up a health food store. With health food and shiatsu as my two major strengths to create positive, life-enhancing change, I thought Philadelphia would be the first of many cities that would be receptive to the idea of promoting and supporting alternative healing centers and modalities.

As Gandhi said, "You must be the change you wish to see in the world." Day in and day out, I was seeking excellence and harmony. By following that kind of thought process, I found my calling, 44 years in the making, and it took a freaking headline to nail my soul and get my butt moving to help create the world as I saw it, with intense drive and purpose. At 44, having a wife, four kids and a successful business, I became passionately imbued with a sense of purpose, which 21 years later still drives me to heights I never dreamed would be possible, making this purpose a viable reality to some extent.

As always, I let things flow into formation. I knew nothing about health food, obviously, since I was a meat, soda, candy and coffee consumer! I knew nothing about supplements as I, personally, saw them as a waste of money. I knew nothing about owning a store, let alone what it would take to open hundreds of them. The exact number I wanted to open up was 240 stores. I thought that each store should try to influence 100 people to speak their truth, and then these people would influence 100 more people.

By my calculation, based on the 240 million people on the planet at the time, that would represent 1 percent of the population. An additional 4 percent, at the time, were vegetarian. This meant that if the 1 percent was added to the 4 percent, or vegetarians, change would occur, I thought. In my readings, I recall that if the population reaches 5 percent of a certain thought process, that thought process grows exponentially. This would negate David Duke's vision of how he saw the world to be. In my infinite wisdom, I had the solution. To this day, as I write, I am still clear that change on that scale can happen. I am also clear that to create the changes we want, we have to be the change we want to experience. It is the basis by which I live and work.

Every cell in my body went into forward motion. I realized I had to change my thought process connected to David Duke. I became transfixed with that notion. I sensed that the tools and knowledge of how to make plans all work would enter my life as needed. At the time, I was a meat eater. At the time, I did not exercise. At the time, for whatever it is worth, I was a couch potato who worked as a deliverer of snacks, coffee and soda.

David Duke's words became my sword for change. I sensed that the following is what I was guided to do: I thought that if I could encourage people to heal their bodies, they could heal their minds and, as a result, heal their negative, dark inclinations. I created a change in five months by becoming the owner of a health store called Arnold's Way. I, who knew nothing about vitamins, herbs or anything connected to health, got into the health food world. I realized I had to find a partner who knew about vitamins and, more important, needed to find someone who knew how to run a health food store. This person needed to be willing to work 60 hours a week for low pay. Fortunately, I was able to find this person. I found my partner after being rejected by at least 10 people. I found the location, and everything fell into place as it was supposed to be. We opened for business in February 1992.

Business was slow but steady. I chose Manayunk, a neighborhood of Philadelphia that was on the cusp of being the new hot spot. Manayunk offered the greatest potential for me to meet the most influential people, who are the leaders making change in Philadelphia policy. The only one flaw in that logic was that, at the time, I had no knowledge of what to say, what to do or even what to think in regard to people's health. I was living a dream. I needed to find the core of my passion and discover precisely what my truth was, and I had no idea where to begin searching.

All that changed very dramatically about three months after opening Arnold's Way. This means that all my hopes and desires and everything that I ever wished for came to a grinding halt. Shortly after my 45th birthday, I suffered many episodes with extreme heart pain—something no man or woman should ever have to endure. I experienced massive chest pains, which were like stabbing daggers. I thought I was going to die right then and there. I had this heaviness in my chest that would not go away. At night, my two little fingers would go numb on and off the whole night. I rubbed them so that I could regain circulation in them. I did not know what to do, but I, who just opened a health store and needed to be a shining example of health for millions, had to face the reality that I might not be alive for my next birthday. I knew from my shiatsu experience that what I experienced was not good.

At the time, I believed there was nothing I could do but wait it out until I found a solution. I began asking everyone who appeared to be in the know, "What I should do?" The stock answers were herbs, vitamins, Reiki, or hands-on healing, or massage. I was panic-stricken and felt somewhat out of control. I began taking special vitamins but to no avail. I began taking special herbs that were supposed to heal my affliction. Everyone thought they knew what would cure me, but no one really knew how the body works and what it is supposed to do.

What holds true back then, 20 years ago, holds true even more today. We, as a people, are inundated with quick-fix solutions such as taking pills or told to go for invasive surgical procedures. We, as a people, are literally scammed into thinking that the body makes mistakes in creating a toxic crisis of elimination and that the crisis has to stop immediately before it spreads.

I was in a panic. I had chest pains, numbness in my fingers, hands and arms to the point where I was afraid to go to bed because I thought that I might not wake up. The only thing I thought would help me was to take a pill. At that time, not knowing anything compared with what I know today, the idea of taking a pill simply did not make any sense. How does the pill know where to go and what to do and how to react? I was told it does and to just take it. So I did just that. I began taking about seven supplements daily, all to no avail.

For two months, I continued in this obsessive manner, depending on an outside force without taking any internal responsibility for my health. I still experienced chest pains. One day, my chest pains became so bad that I told my daughter while driving her to school that I could not take her because I was having a heart attack. I thought I wasn't going to make it to the hospital because I thought I was dying. I came upon an intersection, with one way leading to her school and the other way to the closest hospital. I thought about it and thought about it and thought about it. I said to myself, "Should I take my daughter to school and die or go right to the hospital?" I chose to go to the hospital. I told my daughter: "I can't take you to school today. I'm having a heart attack."

I was in a hospital for three days, and doctors couldn't find anything. They said I could have had a ministroke but weren't sure. I left the hospital with chest pains. I also had pains in my left arm and was continually out of breath. I could not walk 20 feet without being out of breath. So one month later, I said to myself, "I'm going to see if I can get better." I didn't know what to do but knew I was doing something wrong. One month passed, and my chest pains did not go away. I said to myself, "What should I do now?" The only thing that came to me at that point was to see my doctor again. He ran an EKG on me and said, "Arnold, you have to go to the emergency room right now."

I went to the emergency room for the second time in one month's time. I did not think I would live to be 46. I thought I was going to die. I was incredibly scared of what would happen, and more important, I knew that I did not want to die. It was under these circumstances that I went into the hospital. At the emergency room, I had to wait for my number before getting examined. They put me in a gown, and I saw all these big machines. I saw all these old people lying down. I saw doctors and nurses running around, and I felt very helpless. At that time, I was married. I told my wife to get me out of there. I told her I didn't belong there. I wasn't ready to die; I had plans to *be* the change.

While I was in the hospital the first time, tubes ran up and down my body. With my wife holding my one hand and with my daughter holding my other hand, I asked myself what I was doing wrong. I felt that I was a hair strand away from death. I decided that I'm going to take full responsibility for my health. My friends, this is the key. I decided that I was not going to depend on anyone else for my health and well-being ever again.

I realized I was not doing two things I knew I should have been doing. I wasn't exercising and eating salads. At the same time, instantaneously, I recalled a book I read 10 years earlier called *Fit for Life*. I recall a page in that book that said rebounding is the best exercise.[1]

I'm in the hospital dying and recall this one page in this one book I read years ago, almost like an epiphany. The doctors at the time thought that I might have had a stroke, but till this day, no one knows for sure. I said to myself, "Arnold, when you leave this hospital, go get your rebounder." I left the hospital and bought a used rebounder for $10. Four months later, I bought another used one. About a year later I finally bought a good one, which I'm still using today. Seventeen years later, I'm still rebounding. I live and die by this rebounder. Later I will explain to you what it is and why I use it.

The cause of all disease is based on the same theory. When you finish reading this book, you should have enough information to make intelligent choices. The first part is love. Our bodies are beyond miraculous. We are walking miracles of life at its finest. And no doctor, no hospital, no pills and no herbs can do more for us than our own bodies' intricate system of healing through homeostasis and purification on a moment-to-moment basis. My friends, I had an eye-opening experience that day I left the hospital. We just have to pay attention to our bodies' language. There is no more intelligent than our internal wisdom.

These are my transitional experiences. Without either of them, I would not be writing this book and driven as I am to this very day.

When I left the hospital, I had a renewed sense of self-awareness. I wanted my life back. I wanted to live badly and had no choice in the matter. I changed my eating habits but did not give up meat at the time because I was not aware of its harmful effects. At the time, I did not correlate that what I ate directly affected my body's overall well-being. The only thing I began to realize was that I needed to add salads and exercise, particularly rebounding, as part of my routine. I was also aware that I was directly responsible for my health and well-being.

On this note, I began studying anything and everything in the health field. I ate anything that resonated with me in my innate wisdom, which wasn't fully realized as is today. I began studying herbs, vitamins, massages, Reiki, One Brain, homeopathy and many other healing modalities. Each modality had value, but none of them struck me with an "ah-ha" moment in which a light would go off in my brain, indicating that I had found the solution! Each modality helps our bodies to become a little more proficient, but each one, I felt, was not the end-all, be-all solution.

It took six years of studying, taking classes, living my dream and spreading the word about how shiatsu is a strong key to well-being when I finally hit pay dirt in my discovery of Natural Hygiene. I struck it rich, once again, almost by accident—it was all part of the journey. Once again, I became forever changed on the day it occurred, and I feel even more strongly in my belief that this is the way 14 years later.

Chapter 5

My Big Awakening
with Natural Hygiene

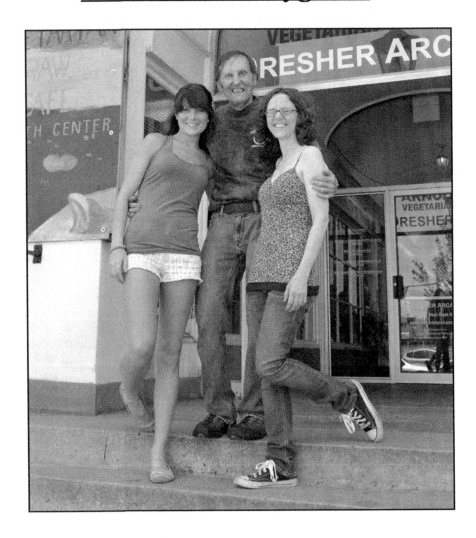

I N THE LATE 1990S, I was obsessed with spreading the word about shiatsu. I thought I knew what my calling was all about but, in reality, I had barely scratched the surface. Still, I was driven by all these promises I made along the way after my David Duke revelation, the energy that stopped me in the middle of a Philadelphia street and the young girl who gave me a powerful insight about what is real and what is not real. For whatever reason, I believe my purpose and mission is to share my journey.

It is from this premise that I was led to open another store called Arnold's Way II. I was on my way to open the 240 stores, but years later, after closing the second store, I realized that dream could not occur, but the vision still exists in my mind. Everything seemed ready. I made the money to open the store randomly on a wing and a prayer. I bought all the vitamins, herbs and extracts to stock the shelves to make the store work. Everything was ready except for one little thing. I was in the wrong mode of thinking. I still was operating from the belief that pills can heal a person. I also knew that I had a higher power as my protector who was guiding me every step of the way.

Within this framework of creating, designing and supplying the store, I had a window of opportunity to take a home study course written by T.C. Fry based on Natural Hygiene. It was a compilation of 14 books that dealt with the process of the body, how it works and how the body is adversely affected when improper dietary choices are made.

I had to read and complete the 14-book course in the two months before opening the second store. What I had intended to do didn't happen, but I opened the store anyway. I finished 10 of the books, but from the very first page, I instinctively knew everything I espoused, taught and served at the Manayunk store just wasn't right. I realized that I was headed in the wrong direction. I was serving the wrong food, giving the wrong advice on what herbs and vitamins to take and felt somehow incomplete in my service to others and myself. I decided to change course and change the way I ran the business.

The true story is that after reading T.C. Fry's first book on Natural Hygiene, I was forever changed in my actions and words. His teachings encompass with the natural flow of life on how our bodies receive, how they interact and how they let go. He talked about a way of living in accordance with the laws that govern our bodies' existences as a path to true happiness.

On the first page, I was so totally impressed, so totally mesmerized and so totally connected to my remembrance of Lucy's statement: "Let me close your eyes forever." After reading the first page, I knew I would be doing a disservice to my customers by selling them vitamins, herbs and cooked vegetarian food. It was not the way of Arnold.

So I opened the second store, but from the very beginning, it was "survival city," meaning I had to work many hours with little money coming in, but my heart and soul was on fire. I instinctively knew that this lifestyle—Natural Hygiene, which is centered on raw fruits and vegetables, or human beings' natural diet—is my true purpose and passion. The other store was not meant to be. I realized I was spreading the wrong message. I was meant to spread the words of Natural Hygiene in an abbreviated form of unconditional love for ourselves and that which exists around us.

Chapter 6

Natural Hygiene: How It Works and Applies

From T.C. Fry's Body of Work

"NATURAL HYGIENE, a simple health system that is in harmony with nature, in accord with the principles of vital organic existence, correct in science, sound in philosophy, in agreement with common sense and a blessing to humankind."

"Natural Hygiene employs strictly natural means for attaining and maintaining ideal health. This means that practices are commensurate with human nature and not what can be found in nature."

"Natural Hygiene means living in accord with our instincts which are still alive and well despite perversions. Just as animals in nature live vigorous, active and disease-free lives while living by their instincts, so, too, will humans thrive in vibrant, sickness-free well-being when they observe their instinctual requirements."

"Natural Hygiene is a way of life and has nothing in common with the so-called healing arts. Natural Hygiene holds that the organism is self-sufficient if supplied with its requirements, that is, fresh air, pure water, sunshine, exercise, wholesome food of our biological disposition, rest, sleep, security of life and its means and over 20 other life essentials as shown herein. Natural Hygiene rejects all drugs, medications and treatments, holding that they interfere with vital processes and are most often downright injurious. Natural Hygiene recognizes the plainly obvious in asserting that only the living organism can heal itself if injured or diseased. Natural Hygiene is, therefore, devoted to teaching people how to live correctly, i.e., to live in accordance with their biological heritage."

Chapter 7

My Philosophy and Understanding of Life: What Works and What Doesn't

Energy Comes from the Body's Wanting Love

THE BODY RECOGNIZES TRUTHS AND LIES. There is absolutely no shade of gray. As soon as we eat any food, the body has to determine whether it has the ability to absorb, digest and eliminate the food. The body also has to determine and how much resources it must use for these processes to occur. If the food is alkaline-forming—all fruits and vegetables are—the amount of energy that is required to take the food from the stomach to the intestine can be determined in minutes. However, cooked food, which is acid-forming, can require 20 to 60 percent more energy to digest the food.

As soon as food is cooked, it becomes acid-forming. This means that the body can't use it as it is essentially considered acid waste, meaning that cooked food is harmful to the body's efficiency. The body then determines whether it has enough energy to neutralize, store or eliminate the food. All human bodies work in this manner. To be in a state of optimum health, one has to eat raw most of the time. If not, one has to be conscious of the fact that every disease and emotional affliction as well as stress and anxiety is caused by the body's reaction to spending too much energy on digestion.

In the more than 10 years I have been giving classes on a mostly raw lifestyle, only a handful of my students have been able to sustain 100 percent raw for any length of time. Most drop out or give up or simply switch to a less-demanding dietary approach and lifestyle.

Food requires energy to digest. There is absolutely no way around that. The body requires calories and nutrients to sustain itself. Giving the body nutrient- and calorie-rich food that takes very little time to digest is optimum. This kind of food gives the body what it truly needs and wants. This is the perfect love story that happens when one ingests the right kind of food. The body has more energy to rejuvenate and heal itself instead of spending much time on digestion.

Food Is Meant to Nourish, Not Entertain

We as a people are caught up in the ideal of being entertained by color, experience, culture, media marketing, childhood eating experiences and teenage and adult peer influences on what should be eaten, why and when. I'm not saying all this is good or bad—it just is what it is. It must be said that the minutes that should be used for keeping our bodies in a state of excellence are spent eliminating cooked foods.

Almost 100 hours of digestion time are required to eliminate each cooked meal, and that, my friends, is the major cause of all diseases. Every time we eat meat, chicken and fish, we are experiencing the death of that animal, in essence. Every horrific thing the animal or fish experiences while being tortured and killed, we experience. My friends, on a cellular level, our bodies get angry and depressed and literally want to expel this waste residue out of themselves or store it in a very safe place until our bodies can properly do their job.

Every Moment Is a Loving, Caring Moment

What we eat also plays a major role in how and what we think, how we react and how we operate on all levels beginning from the time we rise each morning. What we eat affects whether we are sluggish and barely able to get up or thankful and in humble appreciation for life and being alive. If the food we ate last night is still rumbling in our system, causing dissatisfaction and grumbling, then we are in trouble. If the reason for these reactions is due to the fact that we've just eaten a dead animal, this can cause some serious digestive issues. This waste needs to be eliminated or stored, depending on how much energy the body has available. If the body chooses to store the waste, in all seriousness, it will store it as fat. This is because the body has no choice in the matter given that it requires too much energy to break down this food.

My friends, our bodies call us to be in a state of love. I cannot accept the way meat is processed in this country. Some guy you don't know destroys a live animal, cuts it up into tiny pieces, puts dyes and perfumes on it so it doesn't turn purple or rots when packaged, and then that dead piece of meat goes to stores looking good and fresh in neat packaging. This, my friends, is not love. Every moment is an opportunity for us to live in a space of love. You be the judge. Do you think that being in a state of love means that you kill something, cut it up and then eat it? Our cells understand what is true for the body and try to eliminate or store that which is not good for the body. This is what we call sickness and disease.

Truth Always Overrides

As we live, breathe, understand and walk our path, wherever that may lead, there exists, on some level, no matter big or small, a voice of consciousness that becomes our guideline for choosing which direction to go. As we make better dietary choices and our bodies begin to be freed from being clogged with gook, that truth which enables us to walk, talk, see, hear and breathe becomes stronger in enabling each of us to determine our truth. We begin to gain that understanding to do the body no harm. Otherwise, the body will begin to degenerate at a speed much more so than we desire.

Sickness Is My Strength

Seeing sickness as strength is a hard concept for most to understand, especially in a society that focuses on treating symptoms and not the cause. As I see it, most, if not all, people go into panic at any sign of fever, cough or illness. They imagine these symptoms are not normal and should be remediated right away. They think the symptoms are caused by a bug or virus getting into their systems, causing their bodies either to exert an eliminative action or a conservative reaction as a direct result of all of these millions of viruses attacking the body.

As far-fetched as it may seem, to my knowledge, all viruses are dead and have no communication with one another. It is the accepted belief that the virus causes all these symptoms. Our medical establishment tells us how to identify the beginning of a cold, how it will end and how mucous secretions are supposed to look when the body eliminates them.

The basic belief is that the body does not know what it is doing and that everything is happening from an outside source, including the cold, fever, aches and pains. A Natural Hygiene approach tells us that everything that happens in the body is by the body's design. If sickness or healing occurs, it is because the body is overloaded with toxins and waste. To operate more efficiently, the body decides, to its maximum capability, which is the best method to remove the toxins—through fever, cough, cold or to destroy the toxins by simply isolating them. Then the body uses its own natural healing forces, which are genetically built into our system, to neutralize and remove the toxic waste. It is these forces, called our immune system, that prioritize and choose the best natural option.

If it weren't for these offensive actions started by the body's immune system to heal, mend and remove toxic waste, our bodies could end up much worse. We could even die.

What Can I Do for Others?

For whatever reason, whether good or bad, my lifestyle of eating mostly fruit and leafy greens has created a thinking process that doesn't focus on my well-being but on my being of service to others. It's all about the love, promise, dream and passion. It's the day-to-day mundane routine that is my shining light in a business that focuses on health and well-being. So with my light, I am honored to share with you my path so that you may find your light. It is my belief from the deepest part of my truth that each one is truly our brother's keeper. What prevents us from creating that reality are the dietary habits that reek of death, glue and chemicals, written on the backs of boxes of food. Once these dietary habits are removed, the light within begins to shine much brighter.

Chapter 8

Intelligent Choices
for Better Health

THERE ARE TWO REASONS –and two reasons only—why some choose to stay raw and healthy:

- **Knowledge:** taking total responsibility for our health and educating ourselves
- **Consciousness:** becoming aware of and trusting our innate healing abilities as well as proactively supporting them

These two reasons, based on Natural Hygiene, drive my choices on any given day. It is one of those things that requires a daily commitment to excellence. We live in a kind of world where we are inundated with so many food choices and so much variety. Where do we begin? Where do we end? I rely on my knowledge, which took years to acquire, to make a conscious decision that I will not eat bread, meat or any processed foods. We are confronted with tough choices on a moment-to-moment basis, but once you are convinced of the truth and realize the potential for hazardous consequences, it is easy not to be influenced to sway off the chosen path.

As you walk down any street in America today, you'll observe that more than 60 percent of people are overweight. It boggles my mind that people my age can barely walk—let alone run—when they go someplace. They can't run up steps. At 65 years old, you should be able to run. At 65 years old, you should be like a rocket. At 65 years old, you should dance all night long. You should not be on medication. The basic assumption is that medicine will help a person. My thinking is, "How does the medicine know where to go?" You've got 98,000 miles of arteries. "How does the medicine know where to go?"

I am 65 years proud and still looking forward to the notion that my best and most productive years are to come. I am constantly reading about the importance of food and gravitate toward books that bring this point across. I understand that every minute counts and that the choices I make in life in relation to diet can have major implications in the days, weeks, months and years to come. So, my friends, go forth, increasing your knowledge and enhancing your consciousness.

Chapter 9

My Writing Begins Anew

MY FRIENDS, THIS IS WHAT TRANSFORMATION is all about. This is how my own transformation began in summer 1972. This is how I got to see what is important and what is not. This is the story about how my mission came to be what it is today and that which I feel a need to share with you.

Once again, in summer 2011, for whatever reason, a transformable change occurred. I started to shed my old thoughts about what the body needs to get well and maintain its well-being like getting rid of old, worn-out clothing. I was getting rid of the old and bringing in the new. Just as flowers begin to bloom and fruits begin to ripen, I awakened to a new way of thinking about health and well-being as I shifted to a more natural approach. This summer, though, everything became accelerated in the course of 30 days. Everything I ever considered in my wildest dreams was being crammed into my soul like a runaway train without brakes.

All this began innocently enough without even a tinge of awareness that something really big was about to happen. On June 1, I received an email from Joy King. She inquired about a room to rent, and I happened to have one. I replied that I had a room but that I required one month's rent and one month's security deposit to be paid. She did not answer right away, asking me to give her two days. Within two hours, my friend's mother needed a place. However, I already knew I had already given it to Joy. Joy was going to be my queen muse who would inspire me to achieve my next stage of transformation.

I am not sure why I am telling you all this, but life works in funny ways. I am fortunate enough to trust my inner voice, love for life and passion to determine what works for my highest good. If I were motivated by monetary success alone, I would probably be retired by now, living with the standard variety of aches and pains usually associated with a man of my age.

Living a life without the awareness that every minute is precious and that every chance meeting with someone offers a gift of inspiration to expand your inner vision of who you can be and what you can do isn't really living at all. It's not me. It's the continual pursuit of truth that keeps me driving forward and living from the place of light rather than darkness. It is under these circumstances that Joy moved in. She was originally from Portland, Oregon, and wanted to have a fruitarian-lifestyle community experience. This is, of course, what I am all about. In the same vein, we opted for trade in regard to food. All was agreed upon, and everything changed within a week for both of us. She got a good-paying job, and I provided her food in exchange for her help in typing a book I had begun to write.

I hadn't written a word in more than four years. My drive to write was shut down. I got lost in the computer world. I was overwhelmed and underskilled with computers to write articles and books.

I lost my drive to continue writing articles, which I had previously done weekly for almost three years. I lost too many articles and spent too many hours typing, reviewing and proofreading and then losing them on my computer. It was more of a loss than I could bear. I literally was fried because of all these computer failures. It was on an article about love that I stopped. Since then, every week and month, I desperately wanted to renew my interest in writing. I was not ready until that magical moment when Joy King came into my life.

Truth be told, she provided a jumpstart, inspiring me to begin writing again. The decision to do so was heightened for me about three weeks later, when a businessman approached me to explore the possibility of opening Arnold's Way franchises across the country. It is under these circumstances that I had no choice but to tell my story, explain my philosophy and make clear what drives me to do what I do seven days a week.

When I began to write again, I initially thought that the second chapter, which centers on the nuts and bolts of a raw fruitarian lifestyle, would be the most important. But as I dived into the formation of this book, I realized, like watching a man climb a ladder to a higher rung of achievement, I felt moved to go in another direction. I think if one is strong enough, he or she can make a difference. I think if my passion and desire to succeed is strong enough and I keep the focus on living from the highest place possible within me, then the highest good for all concerned will be realized. Others will not only be inspired to follow in my footsteps but, more important, they will join forces with me to share the dream with others.

A big part of my philosophy comes from the Natural Hygiene approach, meaning that the body has an innate wisdom and intelligence that enables all organs, systems, cells and synapses to function optimally. All the body's processes, according to this philosophy, work together harmoniously without making a mistake from the time of birth till the time we take our last breath.

Natural Hygiene, in my belief, ranks as the highest form of definition for explaining what creates and supports optimum health and what creates and causes disease. There are many paths with many different opinions. Every person makes a decision as to what path is right for them based on whatever one believes at any given moment in time. But when new information is provided and acquired, one's viewpoint can change in accordance with that new insight.

It has taken me almost 40 years of searching, living, adjusting and re-evaluating to know what works best for me.

Chapter 10

Seven Steps
to Optimum Health

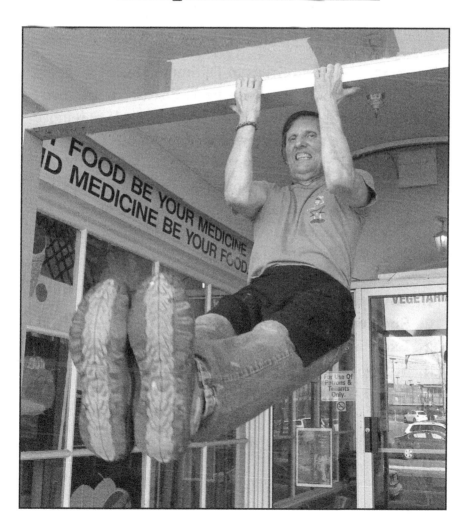

> **"Love" by Arnold Kauffman**
> *The wind gently blew*
> *The sun set*
> *We see the harmonic flow—as the grass sways to the movement of life*
> *Couples hold hands—to grasp the other—for their safety, for their love*
> *Neither wants to let go*

THESE ARE MY SEVEN STEPS to Optimum Health. It is my opinion that only the body heals disease. If the body cannot heal, then it cannot be healed. The secret is to remove the cause and give the body the proper conditions for health, and the body will do everything in its power to start the detoxification and rejuvenation process. The seven steps are written in order of importance for healing to take place.

To cure any disease, no matter what the disease is, you have to follow these seven steps:

1. **Love**
2. **Species-Specific Diet**
3. **Exercise**
4. **Sleep**
5. **Fresh Air and Sunshine**
6. **Water**
7. **Fasting**

We can experience many kinds of love, but the kind I want to focus on is the love needed to heal the body and keep it in the highest state of health possible.

1. Love: Our bodies understand thoughts. Every moment is a moment of love.

The first step is love. We need to be in a state of love. You have 75 trillion cells working in unison. They want to be in a state of love at all times. These cells work together synergistically as an organism representing our bodies, and they never ever make a mistake. This means that your right hand does not hit your left hand and that your right hand doesn't smack your head. There are no accidents. Everything is based on love. For all the 75 trillion cells contained in our bodies, each cell has 20,000 life units in it. That's 150 quadrillion life units inside our bodies working every single day to make sure you're happy. The body wants to be in a state of love at all times.

What does it mean to *love* the body? To love the body means to leave no carbon footprint, or no trace of toxic waste, chemical or residue that forces the body to use its energy to break down and eliminate through whatever channels it deems possible. It also means the body should use the least harmful method for obtaining optimum health performance. It is pure love to the body when we eat a diet that consists of mostly fruits and leafy green vegetables. Because fruits and leafy greens are easy for our body to process, this, my friends, is *love*. Fruits and leafy greens are also alkaline-forming, and this means our bodies require only 40 percent of our digestion energy. When we are on the standard American diet of processed foods and meat-based products, which can stay in one's system for hours, if not days, rotting and fermenting, it takes 60 percent of our energy to digest this type of food. The more energy required to digest the food, the longer it takes the body to rejuvenate and detoxify itself.

2. Species-Specific Diet: We should eat mostly fruits and leafy greens juiced, blended or whole.

The body recognizes truths and lies and never makes mistakes. The same intelligence that determines our births and deaths and the way we see and walk is the same intelligence that determines our vibrancy toward life. If food is good for the body, this intelligence rings true. This means the body recognizes that the food is alkalizing and, therefore, doesn't create any acid residue. As a result of this insight, I became a mostly raw fruitarian.

I eat anywhere from 15 to 25 pieces of fruit a day and most of it in liquid form such as in smoothies or juices. In juice form, the recommended limit is eight to 10 ounces per hour—more might result in blood-sugar issues. If the food is a lie, I will not eat it, almost all the time. The food is a lie if the food is of no use to the body. The life force of fruits and vegetables is broken down and becomes unusable—destroyed, even—as soon as food is cooked above 105 degrees. This means the food is void of all or almost all life-supporting nutrients and becoming denatured vitamins, minerals, enzymes, fiber, essential fatty acids, water, glucose and protein and is no longer raw. These are the nine essential qualities, which are necessary for the body to absorb nutrients from the foods that are put into the body for the body to not only experience optimum health but sustain itself. The body's survival mechanism kicks in, readjusting every cell, tissue and organ to take the acid waste and dispose of, destroy or contain it somewhere in the body. That, my friends, is called disease.

I had a woman say to me, "What about those amino acids?" She was a scientist, about 55 years old and was losing her hair. She was worried about amino acids, and in the meantime, she was eating all dead food. I asked her what she ate. She said she ate rice and beans. Rice and beans! To repeat, as soon as you cook a food above 105 degrees, it's dead. We as a people cannot survive optimally if the major part of our diet is contrary to our well-being.

So what do I eat? Some call it the 80/10/10 program, which is based on fruits for carbohydrates, protein and fat, eloquently described by Dr. Doug Graham in his *The 80/10/10 Diet*.[2] He calls it the "species-specific diet."[2] The reason I've been eating mostly fruits is because this food takes 15 to 20 minutes for the body to digest, and the less energy spent on digestion, the more energy the body has. Even if the average person did absolutely nothing, he or she would use 30 percent of their calories just to maintain his or her basic metabolic rate.

The average person on a standard American diet, or SAD, requires 60 percent of his or her calories to go toward digestion, meaning that every time you eat meat and rice, every time you eat cheese, a donut or bread, all that food has to be broken down. This process requires energy so that the food can flow through our systems in some kind of usable form. The body requires about 30 percent of its energy for basic metabolism and 60 percent of its energy for digestion. Very little remaining energy is left for personal use. Because fruits require little energy for digestion—maybe 30 to 40 percent—

the body now has more energy for personal use for detoxification and rejuvenation.

Four factors determine the best food for health, as quoted from a flier I distribute at my café:

- **Was the food grown in nature?**
- **Was the food found on a tree, bush or vine or the ground in its raw, organic state?**
- **Is the food yummy to the tummy? Can it be eaten in large quantity as a single meal?**
- **Is the food combined appropriately for optimal digestion?**

Before I choose anything to eat, food must be based on three factors:

- **It has to be grown in nature.** Anything you eat should be grown in nature. We're genetically designed to eat foods grown in nature. We're not genetically designed to eat foods that have been processed, cooked and killed. We're not genetically designed to eat foods that have raised in such a way that we cannot eat a large quantity of it. These are the laws of our body, which will remain that way from the beginning of time till the end of time. It's that simple and pure.
- **It has to be grown on a tree, bush or vine.** I'm sure I'm going to get some arguments with this factor. In fact, I've gotten into some arguments about this factor. If a food's not grown on a tree, bush or vine, then I don't eat it. The majority of my food choices are

based on this premise that the food should be grown on a tree, bush or vine.

- **It has to be yummy to the tummy in a raw state and able to be eaten in a large quantity.** Asking yourself whether a food is yummy to the tummy means asking yourself whether you can eat a large quantity of the food as a meal. People ask, "What about ginger?" I challenge anyone to eat ginger in large quantities. No one can do it. "What about garlic?" I offer the same challenge with garlic. If people cannot eat a food in large quantities and it is not yummy to the tummy, then it shouldn't be eaten. That's one reason I never eat broccoli and cauliflower. They're not yummy to my tummy, meaning they don't digest well. For the most part I eat mostly fruits because they're yummy to the tummy.

People always ask me, "What do you eat?" If you follow these three factors, it's very easy to decide what to eat.

On a daily basis, I follow a mostly fruit routine. First thing in the morning after working out for 30 to 120 minutes, I eat mostly fruit. From 4 a.m. to noon, I focus on eating only fruit. The reason I do this is because I have come to understand that we have something called a circadian rhythm, and this means that from 4 a.m. to noon, our bodies are in elimination mode. During this period, the body has a built-in self-cleansing process that has to be honored. The idea is to keep the amount of energy used for digestion to a minimum, meaning just eat fruit because it digests in less than an hour.

Also, in my case, I like to eat a certain amount of calories. This means that by the time I start to eat my first meal about 10 a.m., I need to consume a lot of calories. A banana is about 100 calories. The average person's breakfast should be about 700 calories. What does that mean? It means eating six to eight bananas at a time. That's 600 to 800 calories as my first meal. One banana does not cut it.

People ask, why eat mostly fruit? Why eat mostly apples, bananas or oranges? I ask them why *not* eat mostly fruit? And how many do they eat? If they say "one," that's 100 or fewer calories. If you just worked out for an hour and a half, your body needs a tremendous amount of energy to function. Only giving it 100 calories does not work. I tell people to eat 600 to 800 calories a meal. People say that they'll gain weight if they consume that many calories. If you eat that many calories from eating fruit, I assure you will not gain weight. People ask why they should eat bananas in particular. They tell me bananas make them constipated. Absolutely, bananas will make you constipated if you're eating bananas with milk or sugar or if you have rotting food from meat, chicken or fish in your stomach from the meal you ate the previous night. Keep in mind that every time you eat cereal, meat or anything processed, those foods are acid-forming, and the body cannot digest them easily.

The fact is, my friends, that all the packaged foods eaten in this country are acid-forming. Telling people they should eat acid-forming foods that cause acid waste to build up in the body does not sell unless one advertises heavily. Almost everyone in this country has been duped into believing this strong craving for pretty cereal boxes, whose products contain, essentially, acid waste, which the body can't process.

This packaged cereal, in reality, leads to excess weight, which our bodies do not want. All cereal is C6 H10 O6. Imagine serving your child C6 H10 O6 for breakfast.

Dr. Norman Walker's *Become Younger* tells us that the body can't break down C6 H10 O6.[3] If the body can't break it down, it acts like glue in the system. If it acts like glue in the system, what do you think it does to your thinking? This is why people can't think straight. There are so many things out there that people are mesmerized by and just as cloudy about what's right for them. They believe they should have cereal and milk in the morning. Cereal, though, is C6 H10 O6 and cannot be broken down. The same applies to pasta, rice, donuts, pastries, cakes, bread, etc. The list is so long it's endless. It's like going to a supermarket, walking up and down the aisles, and finding that almost everything can be labeled "acid waste."

Milk is also interpreted by the body as acid waste. Don Bennett writes in *Avoiding Degenerative Disease* that milk contains something called IGF-1, which has been shown to be the key factor in every human cancer.[4] It's a growth hormone found in only two species, humans and cows in identical formation when in pasteurized form. It creates havoc in our bodies, causing all kinds of flagrant chaos to our immune system and is responsible for tumor formation. Bodies are on full-scale military alert, trying to expel acid waste, cleverly identified as cereal and milk, dressed in nice packaging. My friends, we have been duped big time. Milk is at the beginning of the disease process, which results in coughing, sneezing and allergies.

Keep in mind that if cereal cannot be broken down, it has to go through the small intestine. If the small intestine can't break it down, it has to go to the liver. If the liver can't break it down, guess what happens? It starts forming around the waist. That bloated tummy is all that cereal the body can't process. This is all the extra weight you are carrying, and it's converted to acid waste. The body can't use it. The body has to break it down, contain it or eliminate it from the system. When it is contained, this is the fat that you see around your waist, for example. That's your cereal. That was your meal. That was what you thought was yummy. In reality, it's your body protecting itself to keep acid waste from getting into your bloodstream, otherwise it will be harmful to your well-being.

It's the same theory for all cooked foods, including pastries. With pastries, you're not eating pastries—you're eating C6 H10 O6. All pastries have sugar. In *Become Younger*, Walker states all sugar has something called acetic acid, which paralyzes nerve cells.[3] An excess of acetic acid looks like multiple sclerosis, lupus and fibromyalgia. How many people do you know of who are affected by those three diseases? If you remove cereal from the diet, guess what happens? Remove the pastries from the diet and guess what happens?

I have a lady who comes to my store at least three times a week who originally had multiple sclerosis, or MS. Most of her symptoms have disappeared. What she began doing is just changing her diet. Two factors are needed to treat any disease. Remove the cause and give the body healthy healing conditions and the body will heal itself. The body wants to be in a loving circumstance at all times. It does not want acid waste. Who does?

The key is that our species-specific diet says we are genetically designed to eat mostly fruits and leafy greens. We are not genetically designed to eat cereal or pastry, or C6 H10 O6. Imagine going to a bakery in the morning and giving your kids a bagel with cream cheese. I'd flip out. A bagel isn't a bagel—it's C6 H10 O6. Bennett's *Avoiding Degenerative Disease* says grain products contain something called opioids.[4] Opioids are essentially opium, making them the hardest thing to get out of your diet. This is why people can't change their diets. I see it all the time. People come to Arnold's Way and say, "I'm going to do this, but it's really hard for me to give up my bread." They're not eating bread—they're eating C6 H10 O6. It's very hard to get rid of. Opioids are like opium, meaning it's harder to get rid of bread than crack.

Eating Breakfast, Lunch and Dinner

Here, I will review what to eat for breakfast, lunch and dinner.

Breakfast

What I've told people in my 10-plus years of giving classes is to eat eight to 10 pieces of fruit at a time. Within three or four days, they stop completely because they think eating 25 pieces of fruit is too much and boring, and the average person is not willing to digest all that fruit. The average person cannot sit down and have eight oranges. In my experience, very few people can stick to a fruitarian lifestyle right off the bat. This is why I recommend adding fruits rather than subtracting foods from your diet. This is why I recommend drinking at least 32 ounces of green smoothies, blended drinks containing fruits and greens, daily.

Green smoothies represent the key factor for maintaining a raw fruitarian lifestyle. The reason being is that you are getting your nine fruits and one of your six leafy greens daily in a predigested state that requires very little digestion. The No. 1 nutritional requirement on this type of diet is going to be fruits, and the No. 2 nutritional requirement is going to be vegetables. These are the top two sources for any nutrients. Do you want to go for No. 3 or do you want Nos. 1 and 2? The thing is, what do you really want? What does it take for you to stay young? What does it take for you to be active? What does it take for you to believe in yourself as dynamite all the time? What does it take for you to be like a rocket all the time?

What Do I Use to Make a Green Smoothie?

The first thing I do is put four bananas into a blender. I know that I'll be questioned about eating bananas again. Why bananas? They taste good. If you don't like bananas, don't use bananas. Keep in mind, there are no mistakes. Whichever fruits you like are the fruits you'll use. I like bananas. I like to eat as many as 10 or even more bananas a day. I also like oranges, pears and watermelon. I eat all kinds of fruit, big or small. Remember this: Food is meant to fuel the body and not entertain you.

Next, let's talk about greens. Greens are considered a food group apart from other vegetables. All greens have something called cellulose, which is hard for the body to break down. It is very hard for the body to extract nutrients from greens because of cellulose. Only when you blend greens at a high speed is the body able to break down cellulose into a usable form. So greens are great in smoothies, and I'm a big believer in blending. If you're a diabetic, you need more greens and maybe less fruit. A key is to make sure your green smoothies taste good. If they don't taste good, don't drink them. The food has to follow the yummy-to-the-tummy rule plus it has to be grown in nature, meaning it grows on a tree, bush or vine. Next, I add chopped Medjool dates.

You can use any sweetener you want as long as it meets three requirements:

- **It is grown in nature.**
- **It is found on a tree, bush or vine.**
- **It is yummy to the tummy.**

You can eat anything you want as long as at least 80 percent of the time, it meets these three requirements. I use dates, apples, pears and whatever fruit is available. I don't put the core of the apple or the pear into the blender. I generally use apple or pear because it adds a double sweet taste. For children, it's one of the best kinds of food to serve, sweet, rich in nutrients and easy to digest. We have so many mothers who come in with their children, who are drinking green smoothies. This, my friends, is almost a mother's milk because you're getting nutrient-dense food in a predigested state. It's the best; it's mother's milk in green liquid form. Ideally, eat only fruits or fruits and greens—as much as you want—as you want from 4 a.m. to noon. According to circadian rhythm, this is the elimination period, meaning very little energy should be spent on digestion. The less energy you spend on digestion, the more time the body has to heal and rejuvenate.

Another key is drinking green smoothies as needed. I would recommend drinking at least 32 ounces a day. I generally graze on fruits and greens throughout the day, meaning I eat all day long. Besides fruits and green smoothies, I eat about one-and-a-half avocados a day, and the rest of the time I eat other fruits, whatever is in season. I eat anywhere from 15 to 25 pieces a day. This means that I consume 1,500 to 2,500 calories a day, depending on the fruit source. I don't have to worry about weight.

Lunch

Lunch should be your heaviest meal of the day, with nuts, oil or avocado. Lunch should be eaten between noon and 6 p.m. I recommend that if you eat nuts, you should eat them with no avocado or have the avocado with no nuts. Basically, I suggest you eat one fat at a time. I need to give a warning here: Nuts are very addicting. The hardest part for a raw vegan is to stay away from nuts as well as spicy foods and eating very complicated meals. The average gourmet meal is loaded with fats and oil to duplicate the standard American meal. It's also loaded with many ingredients that are too harsh for our digestive system.

Dinner

Dinner should be a light meal. You want to prepare your body for the next day. If you're eating a heavy meal containing nuts and avocado, these foods contain too much fat, which requires a lot of energy to digest. For dinner, focus on eating just fruits or veggies. By eating in this way, you won't feel sluggish the next morning. You won't need coffee be-cause your body is using little energy for digestion. Dinner should be free of nuts and oil, enabling your body to have a peaceful and restful night's sleep.

Imagine if 10 people came into a room and started talking to me at once. Imagine sitting down for a meal in the stan-dard American diet. Say, for example, you eat rice or pota-toes. Say for example, you eat meat, bread and gravy. Say, for example, you also eat dessert. In each food item, there are spices and condiments that are more than your stomach can tolerate. It's as if your stomach is having 25 conversations at once. How happy can your body be while having 25 conver-sations at once? How happy can anybody be with so much going on inside? It's like a giant rumbling Ferris wheel that just fell off its axis.

The 5–5–5 rule

All meals, whether breakfast, lunch or dinner, should follow the 5–5–5 rule. It should take 5 minutes to prepare, contain 5 ingredients and cost no more than $5. Keep it simple so our bodies don't have to overwork. I'll explain this in detail in Chapter 17.

Even if you are a raw foodist, these same principles apply, especially if you are eating raw gourmet foods. Raw gourmet foods are loaded with fats, oils and way too many ingredi-ents. For example, if you're eating a raw pizza, you have the living bread, loaded with many raw items. You also have the raw cheese, loaded with many raw ingredients, and you have the tomato sauce, loaded with at least four or five ingredi-ents. That's multiple conversations going on at the same time. How happy is your body?

The secret to eating for optimum digestion and health is something called the monotropic eating method. This means eating one fruit at a time. If you want to stay in top-notch physical condition at all times, the secret is to add fruits into your daily dietary regime, not take it away. You don't have to do it 100 percent of the time, but at least most of the time. In my opinion, you should not eat this way 100 percent of the time, because this would be too fanatical. I don't want to be fanatic. Most of the time, I want to have energy, but I don't want to be a fanatic about my food choices and the way I eat. Most of the time, my diet involves drinking a 32- to 50-ounce green smoothie and eating my fruits one at a time. I want my conversations to be simple for breakfast and lunch. At dinner, I focus on eating fruits or vegetables. Lunch is my big meal. I don't do this every day, but most of the time I eat this way.

In summary, listen to your body. The secret is to just add more fruits into your dietary habits. Drink at least 32 ounces of green smoothie a day. The body will then begin to experience what it's like to be free and in tune with what it is genetically designed to be: happy, free, at peace and in love with life. It will then let you know—in no uncertain terms—when you are not feeding it right. You'll become acutely aware when your dietary habits are not aligned with your true spirit. The symptoms are almost instantaneous. You will become fatigued as your system uses a lot of energy in digesting foods. This creates aches and pains because the body has to isolate toxic residue from cooked food. The body then uses all its defenses to contain or destroy the invasion of toxins into the body. It does this by coughing, sneezing and causing general irritation. All the body signs say that the host of the body needs to take heed. This toxic residue has to be eliminated. By eating a species-specific diet, the body becomes more aligned with itself by being alkaline-forming, leaving no acid residue in the system.

So, my friends, as stated previously, in my opinion, here are recommendations:

- **Breakfast:** Eat fruits from morning until noon.
- **Lunch:** Eat fruits or veggies with avocados or nuts (only two ounces for the day). This meal is the heaviest meal of the day.
- **Snacks:** Drink green smoothies throughout the day.
- **Dinner:** Eat a light meal of fruits or veggies.

Enjoy the ride my friends!

3. Exercise: Vigorous exercise is best in the morning, three to five times a week.

I want to review a few exercises I do and explain why I do them. My rock for exercise is a rebounder. I started rebounding when I was 45 years old. This was not by chance or accident. I was literally in a life-and-death situation. At age 45, in 1992, I had what apparently was a heart attack. I was on death row, laying in a hospital with tubes running up and down my body. At the time, my wife was on one side of the bed, and my daughter was on the other side. The only things I could think of were: "What the heck am I doing here? How am I responsible for winding up in a hospital?" The only thing I could think about was a book I read 10 years earlier called *Fit for Life*. In this book, I read that rebounding is the best exercise.[1] I realized I wasn't exercising. After re-reading the *Fit for Life* part about rebounding, I bought a rebounder the day after I left the hospital and haven't looked back since.

Rebounding is the most revolutionary exercise out there—bar none. First of all, you have a cell that is surrounded by something called interstitial fluid. The function of this fluid is to feed each cell food and oxygen to remove waste. If waste does not get removed, cells die or become cancerous. When you jump up and down on a rebounder, lymph nodes, which are the cleaning system of the body, open, and waste material drains from your body. Bathing does the same thing, and taking a bath is good, but it doesn't compare with rebounding. I'd rather rebound than take a bath any day of the week. In fact, I do just that most days a week.

Rebounding is basically called a "health bounce." I do this for two to three minutes. And then I do some front leg lifts. These are good for your waist. That's why I have a 30-inch waist. For those with a belly bulge, this form of exercise will really tighten you up. Next I do side leg lifts which are good for the love handles. I have a little bit, but not too much. The next rebounding routine is a key component to my exercise regimen, and I do this about 200 times. I jump up about six inches off the trampoline and by doing this, I double my weight. I'm 145, pounds and when I jump up six inches I become 290 pounds. That means every cell in the body is getting that super strength of readjusting its ability to accommodate this extra weight. This means, for the most part, I don't have to worry about gaining weight. I also don't have to worry about losing weight, which largely remains stable.

Rebounding is my rock, and I rebound daily as part of my 45 to 90 minutes of exercise. That is my No. 1 priority the first thing each day. When I get up in the morning, the only thing I care about is exercising. I don't care about my emails, store or friends. I devote time to me and me alone. I take total responsibility for my health.

My second favorite exercise is Ohm yoga. I believe in yoga a lot. It has made a definite impact on my life, and I do it after rebounding, maybe two or three times a week. It's good for strength, aerobics and building up your body. Keep in mind this is what I like and what I believe in. The key is for you to find your favorite exercise. Whatever it is, the idea is to earn your breakfast. Consider making exercise part of your daily routine as you would brush your teeth every day.

This is an example of my morning routine. I recommend that when you get up in the morning, if you are thirsty, drink as much lemon juice and water as desired and then work out. We have hands, torsos and legs—the key is to use them. To have a tremendous love for your body means to stay young by getting and staying fit so you can experience the sunshine of your life on a moment-to-moment basis. It's a day-in and day-out experience of love.

4. Sleep: The best time to go to sleep is two to three hours before midnight and three hours after dinner.

Set the pace for living life to the fullest from the time you awaken till the time you go to bed. For the body to operate at full efficiency, it requires nerve energy, which can be restored and recharged only through sleep. In my opinion, the optimum condition for sleep is to stop eating about 7 p.m. The last meal should either be fruits or vegetables made without nuts, oils or complex food combining. The simpler the food choices you make, the less energy the body needs to use for the digestive process.

If you have trouble sleeping, consider what you are eating to create that sleepless state. Keep a food journal of your daily food intake. Take total responsibility for your health day in and day out and you'll see your body wants to be in top-notch shape at all times.

Nuts are high in fat and protein, and this can not only increase the digestive energy required to process them but rob you of a full nerve energy recharge. Our bodies are highly charged, highly sensitive and always seeking optimum healing conditions. The best time to go to sleep is 9 to 10:30 p.m. In an ideal world, one should eat only raw organic fruits or veggies for dinner. These are my goals and ideals, by which I aspire to live on a daily basis. Sometimes I succeed, and other times I get close. Tomorrow is a new day and start. We strive to always do our best.

5. Fresh Air and Sunshine: Get at least 20 minutes a day, ideally before 11 a.m. or after 3 p.m.

As the seasons change and trees grow, when a tiny seed is placed in the ground, things begin to happen. The sun activates the water to help the flowers bloom, trees grow and fruit blossom. Without them working in perfect harmony, there is only dry sand that slips through the hands like tumbleweeds blown into dust. Having lived in the desert, having seen the changes once water was added, I have seen how a desert for years can be transformed into a Garden of Eden in just a month. I have seen a blanket thrown onto grass, not allowing the sun or water to touch it and witnessed dead grass dead in a matter of just days. We live in a kind of world where fresh air and water are at a premium. When we ignore the benefits of not being in the presence of fresh air and sunshine, we will begin to experience a decline in health and vitality.

6. Water: Drink as needed, preferably not with meals.

The area of water consumption is a touchy subject among all concerned. I say that one should drink as needed. Listen to your body's needs to determine how much is best for you. I personally do not drink any water. I drink 32 to 40 ounces of green smoothies a day, and the source of liquid is filtered carbon block water (about 12 ounces). This is what works best for me. It is for each individual to make their own choice. There is no right or wrong way to meet your water needs.

Most of my daily dietary intake is focused on fruits, which has high water content. I eat 15 to 25 pieces of fruit daily. I eat fruits that contain mostly water. It is my belief that I am getting sufficient water intake from the fruits and, not so much, the vegetables I select to eat.

Every moment presents us with an opportunity to make a decision that will affect the next moment in our lives. Keep in mind that what you choose to do today is based on the knowledge and consciousness that you have at a given time. When presented with new information, insight and consciousness awareness, you may make different decisions related to your body's water requirements.

7. Fasting: Fast 12 hours daily, ideally from 7 p.m. to 7 a.m., and better if longer.

The last part is about fasting. Every day I strive to fast 12 to 15 hours a day. And this, my friends, is the key to treat any disease. My lifestyle and conditions for optimum health are based on these theories. In my opinion, if these theories don't work, then there is nothing that will help you. There is no vitamin, pill, medication or surgery that can help you in all cases except for some accidents such as breaking an arm. In cases of heart attacks, cancer and other diseases, you always have to go back to the basics. I am a big believer in daily fasting. When one doesn't eat for 12 or more hours, this rest gives your body the time it needs to begin to repair, cleanse and rejuvenate whatever it deems necessary instead of putting all its resources into digesting food.

This should be the easiest part of one's daily routine because fasting gives the body the greatest amount of assistance. It's so easy. Just put the knife, fork and spoon down. The secret is eating enough calorie-rich fruit during the day so you aren't so hungry at night. Otherwise, you will go bonkers by eating everything in sight. Fasting means abstaining from all food and to allow the body to rest and rejuvenate. So when bedtime arrives, you technically have had a minimum of three hours since the last meal. Your body is set to heal and recharge for the next day.

Chapter 11

Arnold's Day–In, Day–Out Secrets to a Healthy Lifestyle

THESE ARE THE HIGHLIGHTS of what a typical day is like for me and what I shoot for on a daily basis:

1. Set goals of intention.

I want to stay young without aches and pains and to have a young spirit enabling me to live the dream. I want to feel the sunshine, dance to the beat and focus on my youthful appearance. My mantra is to be a lean, mean fighting machine while on my continual road to optimum health. I use this as the basis for keeping my body lean while I'm on the road to optimum health. I generally eat cooked food two to three times a week in the form of potatoes or grains. I eat potatoes when I'm eating out socially because I like eating them with veggies. Other times, I'll indulge in a grain meal once or twice a week. I live and breathe this mantra of leading a lifestyle in which 90 percent of my calories come from fruits and greens as well as being a lean, mean fighting machine. These are my tools to maintain my eternal youth.

Even at my young age of 65, I continue to move into greater and greater levels of fitness and optimum health. I read, study and try whatever resonates with me the most.

But for the most part, I tend to stick to a lifestyle of mostly fruits and leafy greens and a daily exercise ritual, outlined in this chapter, that helps me strive for optimum health.

2. Focus on what is working.

This is the real deal. No one knows better than you what works and what doesn't work. Living on a diet of mostly fruits and leafy greens works for me. The secret for me is to eat a lot of fruit, anywhere from 15 to 25 pieces per day. If I didn't eat this amount of fruit, I would probably get into eating more gourmet foods, which are rich in heavy oil and nuts and are very prevalent in the raw foods movement. I feel my best when I'm living on high-calorie fruits and low nut, oil and spice intake.

3. Exercise daily.

In this area, I try to continually stretch beyond my comfort zone whenever I exercise. I have learned over the years that morning is the best time for me to work out. I do a combination of stretching, strength training and aerobic exercise over 30 to 120 minutes. I generally opt to take on one exercise that is a little bit out of my comfort zone. At the moment, for example, I'm learning how to walk hand over hand across an 8-foot beam. It may be simple for some people to do, but I'm finding it hard to do at the moment. I don't exercise at night because I need to consume a lot of calories after I work out. It would throw my whole routine out of balance if I worked out in the evening.

4. Write down and review your life goals periodically.

Once again, a lot of what I do is about me and how big my ego is and what am I willing to do for my routine to be maintained.

My major goal is to be happy with who I am and what I'm willing to do to create purpose and unity in my actions and words. I want to be in the state of love in my relationships at my job, with those I know and even with people I do not know. I want to be like a ship that sails on smooth water. That, to me, is the key.

I encourage you to define what it is you want to achieve, write it down, look at it each morning and then *be* the things you really want to be day in and day out.

5. Eat enough calories to maintain your body weight (weight multiplied by 10).

This is one of many random statements I'm going to make about meeting your caloric needs. The basic metabolism rate for getting the right amount of calories for your body is based on how many calories are required to be expended. If one did absolutely nothing but lay in bed the whole day and then went to sleep, the amount of calories expended would comprise one's basic metabolic rate. The formula is to take your weight and multiply it by 10 to establish your weight calorie requirement. In my case, my weight calorie requirement would be: 140 pounds x 10 = 1,400 calories a day.

If I were living a sedentary lifestyle, I would add 400 to 600 calories. If I had a very active lifestyle, I would add 800 to 1,000 calories. In my case, I need 2,200 to 2,500 calories daily. I don't count calories, but I do have a base that I shoot for. I keep no food in my house. I eat five to seven bananas after my morning workout right when I arrive at work. As soon as I get to work, the first thing I do is grab bananas and make a green smoothie with 10 bananas (each banana is about 100 calories) and one head of romaine lettuce to get my daily allotment of minerals, not calories, because there are only about 100 calories in a head of romaine lettuce.

Generally, I drink half the 48- to 64-ounce green smoothie during the course of the day. I like to drink four to 12 ounces at a time and eat five more bananas in addition to the bananas included in smoothies I make. I like to eat 40 to 60 percent of my caloric requirement from bananas. That's about 1,000 calories. I also shoot to have 10 dates, which, at 55 calories apiece, amount to about 500 calories along with celery to add more greens into each day's regimen. I generally eat 1½ avocados to meet my fat requirements.

Using that as my foundation, if I stick to this program, by 6 p.m., I am satiated for the day, happy and content. I don't feel deprived in any way and have no desire to stray from this eating plan. Then I do my dry fast three or four days a week from 6 to 7 p.m. till 10 a.m. the next day. I have been on this routine since spring 2012.

6. Rebound three to four times a week.

Rebounding has been my rock exercise for about 20 years. I literally live and die by this form of exercise as my foundation before anything else. The main reason I enjoy doing this exercise and strongly advocate it is because it helps keep the lymphatic system moving, and this boosts the immune system. Doing this exercise keeps the body young.

Rebounding works on three levels:

- **Acceleration (upward motion)**
- **Deceleration (downward motion)**
- **Gravitational (downward pull)**

When these three parts are joined in a single jump, the lymph system begins a pumping action to remove all water that surrounds each cell. When this happens, the immune system has more room to move, and when it moves, it will attack any cell that is not part of the body, especially cancer cells. These cancer cells are destroyed by one immune fighter in particular, the T8 Cell, which contains hydrogen peroxide. This agent kills all cancer cells that it zaps.

7. Drink lemon juice and water.

Of everything I believe in, this one step is extremely beneficial for the body. Drinking lemon juice is very alkalizing and raises the pH of the blood—plus it starts the small intestine's peristalsis movement. Drink as much as you desire.

8. Earn your breakfast.

This is a big one for me. I believe one can't eat until he or she's earned it. This is why I exercise from about 6:30 to 8:30 a.m. I can't imagine living any other way than starting my daily routine with exercise, loving every moment of it, along with eating mostly fruits and leafy vegetables for the rest of the day. Doing this keeps me going steady on a smooth climb to complete nirvana. I love, thrive and am complete on this routine. Every moment is a blessed moment.

I have eight to 10 different routines that I complete and do a little cardio exercise, a little strength training, a little re-sistance work and any exercise that pushes me out of my comfort zone. I incorporate as many different kinds of exer-cise into my routine as possible. I have a mantra of four words that is imbedded in my soul as I go about my day. This mantra drives me daily, monthly and yearly to maintain my youth and my stamina—and help me be a light for others. These words are "lean mean fighting machine."

I used to exercise in the evening but couldn't get enough calories in to maintain my weight. Exercising at night doesn't work for me because, in my experience, when one eats after an exercise session, this activity causes the digestive system to work harder than usual, causing nerve energy to become depleted. Digestion needs energy to break down, assimilate and transport nutrients to wherever they need to go. When I exercised at night, doing so adversely impacted my sleeping and bodily restoration process. Needless to say, I don't exer-cise at night anymore.

9. Eat only fruits—or fruits and greens in green smoothies—until noon.

This is a big one for me because after working out I am starving. What works best for me is eating five to seven ba-nanas and making a supersize 64-ounce green smoothie with 10 bananas and maybe an ounce of dates and a whole head of romaine. The reason I suggest eating fruits until noon is that the body is programmed by something called the circadian rhythm, which is from 4 a.m. till noon. The body enters an eliminative process, cleaning out all the debris and toxic matter that accumulated the previous day. To benefit the body during this process, keep digestive energy to a minimum. This is easily obtained by eating fruit juices or a calorie- and nutrient-rich fruit or green smoothie that doesn't tax the digestive system.

10. Eat enough calories.

This is one of the hardest things to realize. The body needs "X" amount of calories not only to survive but thrive. Most food served, sold, bought and eaten is calorie-rich but nutrient-poor. To thrive, we need to have calories and nutrients. Vegetables have very few calories and are very low in glucose, which is found in great abundance in fruits. Therefore, fruits should be the major source of calories and nutrients. Eating the greatest amount of our calorie intake between 10 a.m. and 5 p.m. will not only satiate our appetites but give the body enough calories so it won't be hungry at dinner. Dinner should comprise a low-calorie meal of fruits or veggies, and this meal should, ideally, be completed by 7 p.m. or three hours before going to bed.

11. Eat your fat at lunch.

I am a firm believer in a low-fat regimen, as per the 80/10/10 dietary program, prescribed by Dr. Doug Graham.[2] It clearly states that a high-fat diet is the major cause of most diseases.[2] High fat not only blocks the uptake of nutrients but clogs the arteries, slowing the transport of—and making it almost impossible to deliver—nutrients to the cell. All this means is that fat is harsh on the body for processing. In an ideal world, it is best to eat fat at lunch because, according to our built-in circadian rhythm, elimination takes place from 4 a.m. till noon, the reason it's best to eat only fruits in the morning. This kind of food is easy to digest, requiring little energy. Digestion truly begins at noon, the best time to eat your heavy meal for calories and fuel and to give the body enough time to properly digest all food. Assimilation is from 8 p.m. to 4 a.m., when the body begins to absorb all the food taken in during the day. This is the time to stop eating so you won't interfere with your body's natural healing, cleansing and recharging processes.

12. Drink 32 ounces of smoothies every day.

Believe it or not, drinking 32 ounces of smoothies a day is the secret to staying raw for the majority of the people who begin a raw vegan lifestyle. I have been giving classes on raw foods with an emphasis on fruits for more than 10 years. In all these years and of all the thousands of people I have taught lessons in raw foods and Natural Hygiene, only a handful of students were able to stay raw for any length of time. The reason for this is that this lifestyle approach is just too foreign and extreme and not in sync with the American culture. In most cases, up until the introduction of the green smoothie, most people could not continue their raw lifestyles.

For whatever reason, the green smoothie works. It has not only been my salvation but to most of the people to whom I have taught a raw foods lifestyle. Green smoothies are easy to make. Just put all the ingredients into a blender, add water and presto—you're done! Green smoothies also taste great! By adding fruits and leafy greens together, with an emphasis on bananas and dates, they have almost the nutritional value of mother's milk. Wow!

Become Mr. or Ms. Popularity! Make green smoothies for your friends, neighbors, school functions and group functions. Share your secret! People will love them and, more important, they will feel the difference.

Green smoothies are nutrient- and calorie-rich! In society today, most prepared food is calorie-rich and nutrient-deficient. The reason for this is that as soon as you cook a food above 105 degrees, you destroy the life force of the food. Green smoothies are loaded with goodness! This, my friends, is the secret that makes the whole raw foods regimen work!

A Basic Recipe for a Green Smoothie
This recipe makes 32 ounces. Drink at least two 16-ounce servings a day.

- 2 bananas
- 1 pear
- 1 apple
- 1 ounce of dates
- 2 to 4 leaves a greens (kale, collards, romaine, etc. and alternate throughout each week)
- 16 ounces of water
- Love

---

13. Eat fruits or veggies for dinner.

In my opinion, dinner should be the least-toxic load on your digestive system. Most fruits are mostly pure water, taking less than an hour to go from the stomach to the intestines. This time frame also enables the body to have sufficient energy to detoxify and rejuvenate what needs to be repaired first in the body. The same holds true for veggies. The secret is getting most of your calorie requirements from 10 a.m. to 4:30 p.m. Then, from 5 p.m. to 6:30 p.m., the food requirements of the last meal won't be as great, and you won't have any last-minute food cravings and will be totally satisfied after dinner. When this regimen is followed, you are ready for the important stage of sleep to restore your nerve energy. The body is fully prepared to do this while expending only minimal energy on digestion.

14. Stop eating at 7 p.m.

This thought process goes along with fasting and the Seven Steps to Optimum Health, outlined in Chapter 10. If the last meal is either fruits or veggies, which take minimal time to digest, the body, in its infinite wisdom, will continually move toward homeostasis and rebalancing the system from the most-minute organism to the most complex. I suggest that all eating stops at 7 p.m., more or less, and that you eat your first food at 10 the following morning. By not eating from 7 p.m. till 10 a.m., you are giving yourself 15 hours of not eating, 15 hours for bodily repair, 15 hours of rejuvenation and simulating detoxification. This, my friends, is one of the major secrets of staying fit, young and ageless.

15. Open a window.

Our bodies need a continual flow of fresh air and sunshine. When we deny our body the earth life force, we deny ourselves a major source of fuel our bodies require. In the summer, many of us stay inside all day in an air-conditioned environment, replete with recirculated dead air that's loaded with microorganisms, which can wreak havoc on the body's immune system. If we stay indoors most of the time in the winter months, we suffer from colds and flus because we aren't getting sufficient fresh air or sunshine. In my opinion, if either of these seasonal factors bothers you, at the very least, keep your window open.

16. Go to bed early.

Sleep is the body's built-in battery, which enables the body to be in a constant state of renewable energy. Sleep is the power force that keeps all the body's processes moving. If the body desperately needs to recharge and you forcefully try to keep it awake, there is absolutely no contest. The body will win. The most effective time to go to sleep is two to three hours after dinner, meaning 9:30 to 11 p.m., when our digestive energy is quiet and the darkness calls our souls to lie down, close our eyes and become one with sleep. Our bodies are aligned to sleep when the sun sets and awaken when the sun rises. Our bodies have this innate wisdom for perfection and optimum health. Sleep is the cornerstone for creating quality burn of fire that can ignite our souls.

17. Don't beat yourself up.

Life is a long, long journey with many ups and downs, curveballs and home runs. Each challenge represents a beautiful part of the ride. We have to be gracious and accept the ebbs and flows of our lives. This is life. One of my favorite quotes is, "How is this to my benefit and what can I learn from this experience?" This means you can take a negative experience and quickly change it into a positive one. Realize that all those thoughts and feelings that literally suck the life out of us because of negative interpretations can be quickly changed in any given moment to sunshine thoughts.

These are my 17 day-by-day steps, I strive for on a daily basis. These are my daily rituals, which keep me on a continual vacation and enable me to thrive, not just survive. I want to live a life of purpose and not get bogged down by a daily life routine. I feel that at 65, my life is just beginning on all levels. So, I am sharing my path with you with humility and gratitude for your giving me this opportunity. I invite you, my friends, to learn or discard the information I'm providing here as you see fit. The choice is yours.

Chapter 12

Seven Stages of Disease

"The universal basic cause of disease is the body's reaction to an accumulation of toxic material."
—*Herbert M. Shelton*

EVERY DISEASE IS BASED on this one sentence. In the medical field, there are about 4,000 diseases, with most of the diseases listed as an unknown cause. According to Natural Hygiene, every cause is known. The body recognizes truth and lies. There are absolutely no shades of gray.

As soon as you cook food above 105 degrees, the life force of a food is destroyed. This means that when you cook the food, the vitamins, minerals, protein, enzymes, essential fatty acids, fiber and water can be minimally used by the body. The body has to use all its forces to neutralize, eliminate or store the toxic waste. The reason the body does this is because we are genetically designed with a built-in DNA code to constantly rid ourselves of toxic residue. This is the goal of every one of our 75 trillion cells, or life units. These cells continually work together in harmonious flow to create perfection, doing whatever it takes for our highest good to be realized.

The body's goal is purification, re-establishing homeostasis and repair of bodily damages. The accumulation of toxic material is called toxemia or toxicosis. There are seven stages of disease, according to Herbert Shelton, a raw foods pioneer.

Every single second we are alive, our body, through its vast communication system, strives for perfection, harmony and peace. This same intelligence keeps our hearts beating 24/7 without a missed beat and causes us to involuntarily blink our eyes. This innate intelligence enables each of us to speak words coherently or unintelligibly so that the words flow out like lightning bolts in a continual swish of joyful understandable audible sound. My friends, this is what purification and bodily repair is. This body works 24/7 to make every part of your body work at optimum performance. According to the laws of nature, many levels have to be in harmony with the rules that were genetically designed for us to rock 'n' roll till the day we die.

In his writings, Shelton describes to us these seven stages of disease:

Stage 1: Enervation, or Nervous System Exhaustion

This is a condition of an imbalance in the ratio of available body energy relative to the nerve energy available for necessary task performance.

Sleep is the key here. To obtain the best sleep to achieve optimum healing, one needs to follow the natural laws of the body. This means we must stop eating three to four hours before going to bed. Refraining from eating this amount of time enables the body to experience peace because it's not working hard to digest foods. Cooked foods, in particular, make the body use every available resource to digest foods because they take a long time to digest, keeping the body from restoring nerve energy for the next day's activities.

This is why people who get sick are tired and why they are not able to achieve optimum health and performance. An imbalance is created by ingesting too much toxic waste, which our body constantly struggles to neutralize. We need to remember the basis for life is built right into our DNA structure, which has to be honored and blessed. We all need to realize that we cannot overdo anything. We cannot live on less sleep with more noise, too much computer use or excessive running, for example, without experiencing a breakdown.

Continually disregarding the laws of nature creates a gradual physical and/or moral weakening, which, if not corrected, continues to worsen and further debilitate the body. Sleep restores and provides energy to the nervous system, and quality food energizes the rest of the body. The best way to restore nerve energy is to sleep.

The body works like a car alternator. If it doesn't continuously recharge its battery, eventually the car will stop. Amazingly, the body works on the same level. Our bodies require sleep so they can continuously recharge themselves. Similarly, our bodies work optimally when they require a minimal amount of energy spent on digestion. Our nutritional intake requires foods the body can readily accept in a whole, ripe raw organic form that is alkaline-forming. Once a food is cooked, the entire body's workload is increased exponentially, impacting all parts of the restorative process.

One needs a clear understanding that the body is continually seeking to be in a state of balance. If you take one piece of the puzzle away, the body becomes imbalanced. Eating the right kind of foods is important. Getting to bed at the proper time and under the proper conditions is necessary to get a good night's sleep. Getting sufficient fresh air, exercise and love is also a part of the lifestyle puzzle as well. When any of these parts isn't properly implemented—with each part being in harmony with the whole body—imbalance occurs.

Stage 2: Toxemia or Toxicosis

If the body doesn't have the energy to eliminate toxic substances, blood, tissues, the lymphatic system and interstitial fluids become imbued.

As I write each word, I realize that I sound like a broken record. I keep repeating myself. The reason for sickness, health or staying young is so simple. The body has a continual quest to be loved, nourished and cherished and live a life free of waste debris caused by eating foods we are not genetically designed to process.

The toxic materials may be generated exogenously, or originating from outside the body such as through poor food choices or from topically applied toxins. It is important to note that just as the body does not want toxic waste to eat, the same rules apply to salves, lotions, moisturizers, creams, balms, etc. Those pretty bottles with fancy names and beautiful pictures contain a long list of ingredients that are man-made and, if ingested orally, will get you sick. My friends, those same ingredients you would never dream of eating we don't think twice about when it comes to putting these substances onto our skin. These ointments and makeup are absorbed into your bloodstream through your pores within 20 minutes. Where is the logic? Where is the common sense? The rule of thumb is always: If you can't eat it, it shouldn't go on your skin.

Inhaled toxins is a tough subject for me. In the past 10 years, I was really sick twice. The first time when I was sick was at 56 years old. I almost went down. If it wasn't for my strong belief in my innate healing ability and following the basis of optimum health, I would have died. There is no question about it—I was that close. I inhaled toxins from mold in my basement that got into my air conditioner. These toxins then got into my immune system, which was already in a weakened state. The year this happened was the year I lost my eyesight in one eye two months into a new hobby: trying my hand at amateur boxing. I tried to clear the vision problem by doing a lot of cleansing fasts such as a water fast, juice fast, a semi fast and a dry fast. I wound up losing too much weight and then gaining all my weight back. I was actively destroying my body by this yo-yo approach to regain my eyesight. My eyesight eventually restored itself after all natural approaches over a year and half failed.

In my infinite wisdom, at that time, I thought my eyesight could be restored just by doing a fast. I couldn't restore my vision through fasting, however. Over and over, I began fasting, and to my surprise, after each fast, my eyesight was not restored, not even the tiniest bit. I had something called a traumatic cataract, which means that something either hit or poked me in the eye, causing a film reaction by my body, and I lost eyesight in that eye. I elected to go for cataract surgery, which, I swear, took only three minutes—and my eyesight was restored. In any case, the mold was the final straw that almost put me down, with my body being so weakened by all those fasts, which, in the end, did not prove successful.

What I am saying is that if you determine that your house, car, job or neighborhood falls into the category of containing too much toxic residue for the body to handle, get out. It's that simple and pure. You are fighting a losing battle by staying.

These toxins may be also generated endogenously, or originating from inside the body, as in the case of cellular metabolic debris. It is important to discontinue unhealthy practices at this stage otherwise the body will begin to experience irritation.

Stage 3: Irritation

Irritation is the result of the nervous system's detecting an overabundance of toxic material. This irritation may manifest as an itch, sneeze or feeling queasy, jumpy, antsy, irritable and/or aroused, with bodily urges or general annoyance. This irritation is a prodding from the nervous system, signaling distress. This prodding is saying, "Take heed" for if the causes of the toxic material are not discontinued or cleared out of the body and if the body is not rested, the body will then introduce the next stage of disease: inflammation.

This is the natural flow of life. The human body wants to be in a state of love at all times, every minute and every second, and it is on a 24-hour vigil, never resting to maintain perfection for all 75 trillion inhabitants. Together, these inhabitants make up our body.

The body has an incredible, unbelievable supreme fighting force that initially, in the first stage of experiencing irritation, creates a minicrisis to rid the body of excess toxic material and has enough energy to expel it. It does this through any channels necessary—by the mouth through a cough, by the nose through sneezing, by the ears through wax building up, by the body through movement and by the large intestine through diarrhea. The body has an amazing grace of innate intelligence. There are no accidents in the body, which is continually on guard and ever vigilant, doing whatever it takes to rid itself of that which does not belong. What does not belong is called toxic material, which is acid waste residue derived mostly from cooked foods as an internal backup of acid debris. Acid debris resides in the system.

Stage 4: Inflammation

Inflammation is a local response to toxemia and injury on a cellular level. It is characterized by capillary dilation, leukocyte infiltration, redness, heat, fever and/or pain as a mechanism to start the elimination of noxious agents and/or damaged tissue.

Let's look at each word carefully. Let us think back to when we were young—all those coughs, fevers and ear aches and all that sneezing. All those childhood ailments that we experienced, at the time, we thought they had to be stopped. We thought they were a sign of sickness, not health. We thought by taking medication, it was the best thing for our bodies, and by taking herbs, it wouldn't be as harmful because it was natural. It would be the best thing for our bodies to put on a salve or cream. This ointment would soothe and heal our condition, we thought, thereby being the best thing for our bodies. Little did we know then and to this day that our bodies are working feverishly to rid the body of these noxious agents. We thought that by placing a foreign substance in or on our bodies that we would heal the condition. In reality, it does the exact opposite. It shuts down the body's attempt to heal, and the body's energy is transferred to neutralize the foreign substance, thereby reducing our healing energy.

Pain and redness is the body's natural attempt to resolve the challenge. What the body needs is to be rested and left alone so it can heal the pain and suffering. The sufferer has been led to believe by the powers that be that the symptoms are not a natural reaction, but, instead, an unnatural occurrence that has to be stopped immediately. At this stage, the sufferer usually will contact a physician not only for guidance but for results, which usually come in the form of a pill. Unfortunately, the assistance usually given is something that suppresses the cleaning process and further thwarts the body's natural healing process. In fact, medications further increase the amount of toxins the body has to cope with because the body does not recognize foreign chemical substances that have no intelligence or nutrients. Medications are considered foreign invaders and have to be destroyed immediately. When this happens, all symptoms stop because the medication is the greater harm.

We begin to realize there actually is an intelligence that is far greater than we can begin to realize. Inflammation is based on that intelligence to heal. Pain is a loving signal from the body that it is becoming more inundated and saturated with toxic material. In the case of inflammation, which can take the form of such conditions such as arthritis, colitis, tendonitis and more, the individual will often seek medical intervention for a cure, believing prescribed medication, if taken, knows exactly what to do and where to go. How does the medication know where to go? The medication has to travel through 98,000 miles of arteries. This, my friends, is hard to believe. No medication, to my knowledge, has any camera or navigation system to assist it in finding the troubled area.

The theory goes on to say that the medication will not only go to but repair the troubled area. Once again, this seems absurd because anything that is able to be absorbed by the body has to have nine requirements: vitamins, minerals, enzymes, essential fatty acids, water, glucose, protein, raw and fiber. The medication taken has none of these nine essential life-building elements and is looked at by the body as essentially not only devoid of life force but dead material. The public is led to believe medicines will somehow heal, cure or alleviate the body's various symptoms. This is not the case.

The body, with its intelligently developed immune system, is working feverishly to destroy, neutralize or isolate the medicine, called "toxic waste" so that it stays away from the main organs of the body. This acid waste may wind up settling anywhere in the digestive tract as colitis, Crohn's disease, etc. All these diseases and this suffering is simply the body's way of isolating and strategically placing the acid waste so it can send its millions of soldiers to destroy and neutralize the residue, to be passed into the bloodstream harmlessly. This, my friends, is the redness and swelling. This, my friends, is the 24,000 diseases named by the medical field. It simply takes all the body's life force to effectively work and do its job.

In regard to inflammation, the body selectively chooses the area to be expanded and then sends millions of soldiers to that area to destroy and remove the acid waste. In human terms, inflammation demonstrates that the body is effectively working. However, according to the medical establishment, some type of treatment is absolutely necessary to stop the pain. According to Natural Hygiene, if we remove the cause, the body will heal itself. It's that simple and pure.

Stage 5: Ulceration

Ulceration is characterized by the breakdown of mucous membrane or tissue, with disintegration and necrosis (dying) of tissue, often followed by the formation of pus. This is often painful because the nerves may be exposed. The body creates this condition to alleviate itself from an overabundance of toxic material.

As we look at words such as "breakdown," "disintegration" and "pus," we cringe. We don't want to hear, let alone be diagnosed with or subject to, such a condition. However, as we realize that eating cooked foods is not only considered toxic by the body but has to be disposed of in a manner that is not harmful to the body, we begin to understand that if the acid waste metabolic residue is coming in faster than the body can handle, the cells become overly saturated, causing a slow death of the organism. The body is designed with enough vitality and intelligence to know that if this intake continues at the current rate, it will destroy the body to the point that the body may not be able to heal itself. The body, in conjunction with the skin, forces and pushes the toxic waste to the surface as the least harmful alternative in dealing with the toxic overload. Once again, this act is based on love. The body, in its innate wisdom and need to survive, unites in a single force to push the bad guys out of the system.

Excessive buildup of toxins necessitates extreme measures to cleanse. After this has been accomplished and with the cause of the toxicity removed, the body will repair the wound.

Once again, the body knows what it is doing at all times. The body is intelligently designed to do what it needs to survive or thrive from the moment of conception to the moment of death. The body never makes a mistake. Not ever! As long as the conditions of health are present, the body's 75 trillion cells work together feverishly as one singular organism to purify the body and to establish homeostasis. In other words, we have to give thanks to our body for creating the warts, fungi, skin rashes, eczema and psoriasis as a sign of love and hope. The body is actively working for our benefit without a single mistake. So we have to be grateful with how the body selectively and intelligently chooses its method of elimination so that toxins will do the body no harm internally.

Stage 6: Induration

Induration is characterized by a hardening and filling in of empty space, created by destroyed tissue, with fibrous elements known as scarring and encapsulation. This process of encapsulation engulfs toxic materials in a gelatinous, hardened fibrous sac to isolate them from the rest of the body. This stage is commonly referred to as tumor formation. This is the last intelligent process the body will call upon in an effort to protect vital organs before the final stage of disease.

We have to understand not only our body's intelligence but, on a much higher level, God's intelligence or Universal Energy, whichever you are so inclined to believe. Let me say it again: Induration is the process of encapsulation whereby the body engulfs toxic material and places it into a storage container. This is done so the toxic material, acid waste, won't stray into the bloodstream and cause bodily harm. If an overload of acid waste goes into the bloodstream, the body will die. This represents the body's supreme intelligence. All life units know what to do to thrive, not merely survive. They intelligently organize a system whereby all toxic material is directed to this gelatinous, hardened fibrous sac to isolate toxins from the rest of the body so they don't enter the bloodstream.

One way the body expresses love is by forming these sacs or tumors to protect itself from toxic material until the body has sufficient energy to go to this mass and use its immune system fighters to gather the strength, plan of attack and least harmful way to destroy, dissolve and abolish toxic mass from the body. The body has the power to do so when the proper conditions are in place. Sufficient energy rises when the Seven Steps to Optimum Health, outlined in Chapter 10, are followed. Only then will the body have sufficient energy to remove a tumor in the purest, least harmful way possible.

What I am saying is that if someone comes to me after being diagnosed with breast cancer, I let her read the words from the "Seven Stages of Disease," adapted from the work of Herbert Shelton. I want this person to be fully immersed in exactly what the body is doing for her benefit as a sign of love, not by accident. I let this person fully comprehend that the body does not ever make a mistake and that everything being incorporated within her system is based on intelligence far superior to whatever can be dreamed up by man or woman.

Someone once said that "one cell has more intelligence than all of the world's intelligence combined."

We as a people have to humbly appreciate the knowledge, wisdom and intelligence that exist in our bodies from the moment of birth till the day we die. All the body's actions are based on love, the purest form of innate knowing and healing.

Stage 7: Fungation, or Cancer

Fungation, or cancer, is a mutation and proliferation of cells. The cells and tissues go awry due to the disruption of their genetic coding by poisonous toxins. These mutated cells obtain their nourishment from lymph fluid but do not serve the body. It's as if they have forgotten their heritage as human cells with an agenda independent and without regard to the rest of the body. Although this stage is often fatal, if the causes of the pathology are discontinued, the possibility of cleansing, repair and rehabilitation still exists. Remove the cause, and the body is given an opportunity to heal.

When I first read these words, I thought of *The China Study* author, T. Colin Campbell, and about his study involving 9,000 people. Campbell investigated these people's dietary choices and explored what extent their dietary choices had on their everyday existence. Through his scientific research, he discovered that if one partakes in eating meat on a daily basis, the chance of getting cancer is almost 99%. On the other hand, if one does not eat any meat at all, the chances of getting cancer are zero.

So I read about fungation. I read about cancer, and I think about all those people I know with it and all those people I don't know. I think about all those families watching their loved ones slowly disintegrate or be in remission, which the medical community considers a successful state. But remission means that the state of the inactive disease is temporary. It's still there waiting to come back. Imagine having a cough in remission or a fever in remission. Imagine any one of a dozen things in your life that is vitally important and now in remission.

My friends, what I am saying throughout this entire book is that there is a way of living, a way of thinking that is based on the Natural Order of Life, which was given as a gift to us from the day of our birth. This gift needs to be honored, loved and cherished with immense gratitude.

I am in continual humble appreciation for the life I have and my body's intelligence in not only surviving but thriving from my birth till my last day.

This section is dedicated to Susan Amen, who rewrote the complicated words of Herbert Shelton's "Seven Stages of Disease" into an easy-to-read form.

Chapter 13

Do–Inn: Self–Massage

DO–INN IS A QUIET RITUAL I devote myself to doing every day. I look toward performing this practice as a quiet retreat away from the maddening crowd, the hustle and bustle and having to be somewhere at a specific time and getting things done. It is a time when all this madness stops. In this space, I quietly get into a sitting prayer position and just listen to my body's language of being loved and giving love.

It sounds really dumb, but I also do facial massage daily. Every part of your face means something. Every part of your hands means something. Everything means something. All of this knowledge came about many years ago when a young woman said to me, "Let me close your eyes forever." All this passion for sharing information came about through many transformations.

Say, for example, someone walks into my store and is always rubbing his or nose. This is not an accident. Say, for example, I see a young woman who has dark circles underneath her eyes. What I know is that the area under one's eyes represents the kidneys. The black color means trouble. I had no choice but to ask this young woman what she was eating. She was eating a vegetarian diet but a lot of soy. Because she was eating a lot of soy and no fruit, she began to develop epileptic seizures, which she suffered from for two years. She went to the best doctors in the country and not once did any one of them ask her what she was eating. Not once did any doctor ever think to question her as to why she had black circles under her eyes. What I did was look at her eyes and ask her what was going on. She said nothing. Later, she said she had epileptic seizures. I asked her what she was eating and found out she was eating a lot of soy. I asked her about her diet, knowing what I know about facial diagnosis. I said to her that she just needed to add more fruit to her diet and to get rid of soy. She implemented my suggestions, and her epileptic seizures stopped completely. One year later, she was seizure free. It was then that she allowed me to record a YouTube video about how she overcame epilepsy just by giving up soy. This is why I do Do–Inn. It's all about self-love, self-healing and a reason to share.

Head

First, I focus on the head. The head deals with the bladder and gallbladder meridians, which correspond with those internal organs. By doing this exercise, it helps activate regrowth of your hair. I tell anyone who comes into my café who asks me about hair loss to perform this particular massage. Men are especially affected by doing this on a daily basis —it will help stimulate hair follicles. The first thing I ask them is: "What are you eating?" A lot of times, meat consumption is the major factor in hair loss. (See the last section in Neal Barnard's book *Food for Life*.)

Between the Eyebrows

Next, I massage right between my eyebrows. This area represents the liver, one of the few organs that can regenerate itself. Unfortunately, if we eat cooked food, it is hard for the liver to function over time because we're eating dead food. Liver problems will manifest as a line or double line in-between the eyes as a grayish or yellowish color in the eyes. By massaging this area, one sends love and regenerative energy to the liver.

Forehead

Next is your forehead area, which can have three lines. If you have these three lines and they predominate, it means you have elimination, digestion and respiration issues. The lines indicate you are consuming too much water or protein or a lack of water. On a psychological level, these lines deal with social responsibility and how one adapts in the system personally, financially and in relationships. By doing Do–Inn, or self-massage, we make sure each point in our bodies receives a tremendous amount of love. We either rub gently or very hard on each point based on whatever we deem necessary. This is the reason I don't need a massage—essentially I give myself one three or four times a week. Performing this self-massage is a sign of love for myself and what I do. It is also a way for me to offer gratefulness for life as I know it.

Bridge of the Nose

My next massage point is the bridge of the nose. This represents your pancreas., which produces enzymes to break up food. As soon as you cook a food above 105 degrees, it's dead. A body has to make its own enzymes to break up food. It shows up as a line or two in people who overuse their pancreases. Lines are a sign of pancreatic issues or oncoming diabetes.

Eyes

Next are the eyes, which, according to Chinese medicine, represent the liver. The liver is the chemical factory of the body, producing thousands of needed substances to neutralize the toxic acid waste that can cause the body harm. It is also the body's main source for detoxifying and neutralizing harmful substances that enter our bodies. It is the only organ that can regenerate itself. The liver will give outward signs through the eyes that it is on overload by becoming red, inflamed, puffy and squinting—as well as by producing failing eyesight.

On this basis, I place the palms of my hands on each eye, cupping them, keeping my eyes closed. I relax, breathe in, breathe out and feel the reflection on my body, seeking relaxation and peace. As I continue massaging, palming and rubbing whatever is so desired, I pay full loving attention to each part of the body to maximize the healing process.

Whether it is the face, hands, chest or torso, each part of the body acts as an individual unit of the whole. I do not differentiate with their needs. Every square inch of the body needs to be touched and loved. As we live and as we age, if we stray from the basic needs of our bodies, an internal conflict erupts. The body becomes stressed. All the forces become mobilized to form a "lean, mean fighting machine" to destroy, neutralize, capture and remove the enemy. In most, if not all, cases, the source of the problem is cooked food, forcing the body to make a series of decisions to determine the best way to neutralize this foreign invader.

If the body decides to store the foreign invader, it can look like fat, meaning the body's chief detoxifying organ, the liver, has to break up and destroy acid residues that are by-products of cooked foods. If the liver gets overloaded, it sends these acid residues into the cells. If the cells can't break them up, the acid residues are then stored around each cell, otherwise known as fat. This happens at the beginning stages of the body's struggle to handle the offensive substances.

Keep in mind, at every inch of one's body there exists a meridian channel that corresponds to an organ. If there is a mark, blemish, pimple or growth, it is not only a growth on the outside but a sign of a particular organ that is in distress on the inside and feverishly trying to cleanse itself. The body has its own vast source of intelligence that not only continually cleanses itself of all metabolic debris but lets one know in no uncertain terms which organ is taking the brunt of the attack.

By performing self-massage, we reinforce the idea that love of life is derived from the universal power of sunlight, the earth, trees, grass and the animals. Loving who we are provides an extra boost to our immune system. This form of massage provides a means of giving thanks for being alive.

So we continue with our self-massage to give each part of the body love. We all want to be loved and give love—and be in this state of being all of the time. I hear stories from my customers about illness, skin conditions, fatigue and aging. I hear about the aches and pains in their joints, their failing vision and their woes about weight gain. I hear it all. I listen, I see and I understand their concerns. I have a clear understanding that what we eat, what we feel, when we go to sleep and what we breathe into our lungs affects our everyday lives. On a moment-to-moment basis, the body is continually trying to rejuvenate itself as each cell and organ works as a team to achieve purity and excellence.

This book is written by me as an extension of who I am and provides a compilation of what I have studied. More important, I want to share my experiences and transformation in living my dream. My mission statement is: "To create an energetic movement for the transformation to a disease-free world."

Chapter 14

Living the Truth

THIS SECTION IS DIFFICULT in one respect and easy in another to write about. It is difficult because I know 90 percent of all diseases in this country that are labeled with a "cause unknown" by the medical field can simply disappear just when people change their diets. It is also difficult for me to realize that if people only knew about all the horrific things happening to innocent animals for us to have these visually appealing cellophane packages, maybe they would think twice about the idea of eating them for food. I think consumers would literally puke their guts out if they knew. People just aren't aware of all the torture going on and mass killing through beheading going on in our factory meat-processing and -packaging plants. This mass destructive energy appears to be driving us not only toward mass animal extinction but is using up the world's water, land and fuel resources.

As we think and ponder all this, we have to consider how our society accepts this kind of death eating as status quo. What's even more absurd is that our society also ridicules anyone who doesn't partake of these social mores. It is still unacceptable to be a vegetarian or, worse, a vegan among eaters of meat and other animal products.

So I write my little words, notes and thoughts about the one major factor causing almost all diseases in not only this country but in the world and world: diet. What one eats determines whether one is physically and mentally strong as the years pass no matter one's age. What one eats determines whether one thrives or merely survives. What one eats determines the actual reality of how happy, peaceful and harmonious a person can be. If people collectively eat a mostly fruits and greens diet that supports peace, harmony and a joy-filled co-existence with nature, I can only imagine what positive transformations can take place. What one eats will also determine whether anger, depression and mental illness will be part of the daily consequences of their lifestyle.

Once cannot eat dead animals on a continual basis and expect to be happy. One cannot eat something that has been horrifically killed and not be depressed, angry and, in the end, mentally off balance. Eating dead animals destroys the very fiber of our existence, lingering for days, months or years. Our bodies are physically and mentally drained through our continued eating of dead food, which has been further degraded through cooking.

So, I ask you, my friends, what is your health and well-being worth? What do you really want and how much are you willing to give up for the purposes of attaining excellent health?

Let's say, for example, people say they can't give up meat. People say they've got to have meat. I hear this all the time. Let's see what meat represents. I've got my friends with me. This, my friends, is called meat. This can be anybody's pet. It can be Charlie, Skippy or Poco—a cat or dog, for example. We think of cats and dogs as our friends. These animals are our loved ones, but what American society does is distinguish between one kind of animal they consider a pet and another kind of animal they consider a source of food. They kill Charlie if it is a cow and eat it.

If I killed my dog, Charlie, and ate it, I'd go to jail—no questions asked. I'd be considered a murderer of the worst kind. I'd be spat on and cursed in total disrespect by almost everyone. People would celebrate my easy conviction by going out to a restaurant and eating a steak sandwich, hamburger or any other meat entrée found in practically all restaurants. It boggles my mind to see the disharmony and contradiction in how little life is worth in the name of eating.

Eating animal and cooked foods creates harmful acid waste that creates havoc in the system and plays a pivotal role in almost all diseases. Let's take a look at cancer. All meat contains uric acid, a known carcinogen and powerful acid. Uric acid is a fancy word for an animal's urine. If it gets near your heart, you die. Uric acid is such a powerful acid that it could destroy our living tissues. Our body understands this. So as soon as uric acid comes into our system, the body has to neutralize it with calcium, derived from our bones or in our blood. Calcium is a mineral that buffers uric acid, becoming calcium uric crystals.

Every time you eat meat, you're eating cow urine. Every time you eat chicken, you're eating chicken urine. Every time you eat pig, you're eating pig urine. Every time you eat fish, you're eating fish urine. Does that speak of love? The body, just like our inner being, requires food that is kind to it. When the body comes in contact with uric acid, it tries to protect itself from being harmed and converts this uric acid into less harmful matter called calcium uric crystals.

The body does not want another animal's urine. Day in and day out, we as a people are eating cow, chicken, pig and fish urine. The body cannot break this down, in my opinion. This behavior, my friends, has to stop. We are not only destroying ourselves, we are killing animals at the rate of millions a day and destroying our world's resources. All this affects the world's ecological system.

The body's basic goal is to achieve homeostasis and balance. When uric acid is in the body, the system needs a special enzyme called uricase. Man is the only animal that does not have this enzyme. The body releases calcium from the hip area in the form of calcium uric crystals to neutralize this uric acid, which cannot be allowed to get to the heart. The body pushes it as far away from the heart as possible. The body pushes uric acid to the hands. This is called arthritis. The body pushes uric acid to the feet. This is called gout. The body pushes uric acid to the back. This is called low-back pain.

Every disease is based on the same theory. Remove the cause. Give the body the proper healing conditions. The body will do whatever it can to heal itself.

The body wants to be in a loving, caring state. The body wants you to eat a species-specific diet. It needs to take in mostly fruit and leafy greens. Add more fruit and leafy greens to your diet. Remove the cause and get your body into a healthy healing condition. Your body will not only heal itself, but the very nature of your presence will vibrate with resounding health exponentially, creating the glow within and to those around.

Chapter 15

Recipes

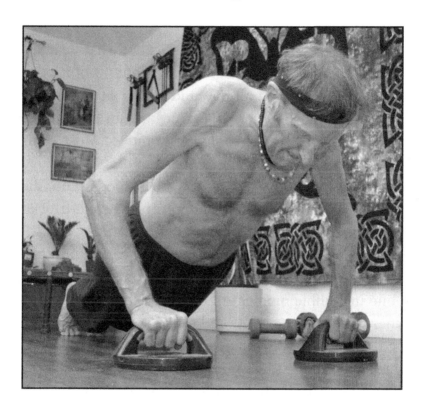

T HIS IS THE HARD PART for me because I am not a recipe guy. The reason I'm not into making complex recipes is because, in my opinion, we are genetically designed to eat whole, fresh, ripe organic fruits in their simplest forms. I like to eat foods that require little or no preparation and that look and taste good.

Recipes

I personally do not believe in recipes. Most of what I eat, as I have already mentioned, is composed of about 90-95% of my daily food intake. I graze all day and rarely sit down for a meal. If I do go out, I generally eat Vegetarian fare such as rice or beans or grilled vegetables or potatoes. Most of the time, I stay away from bread and soy.

In an ideal world, we need to eat the best food for our dietary needs. This means eating a monotropic, or one-fruit-at-a-time, diet is the ideal way to eat, in my opinion.

This is a major component of my daily eating program. This essential component is where it all comes together for me in one incredible moment of utter perfection. This is the part where everything I know and strive and live for joins in one big ball of energy, love, joy and being in the moment of sunshine and total bliss.

Most of my daily dietary regimen is based on eating one fruit at a time. Ideally, I shoot for eating my first piece of fruit at 10 a.m., which is about 15 hours after my last meal. Ideally, I strive for this routine daily. It's my goal and works best for me, but many times I don't get to eat this way. When I step out of this practice for whatever reason, I enjoy the moment and pick myself up and get back into the groove again. That's life.

The logic behind this thought process is based on love. The nature of who we are is based on the love we receive from above, all around us as well as from within. Every breath we take and moment of hearing, seeing and talking come from a powerful source unbeknown to us. It is a plan beyond miraculous. What I am trying to say is that our bodies and all of nature in this world desire and want to be in perfect condition so they can thrive. Our body's goal is to be in a state of continual balance of homeostasis and absolute harmony. If the perfect conditions are not present, then every creature, plant and human being is genetically designed by a higher power with a built-in healing force to right itself or adjust to conditions.

In an ideal world, every bird, plant and human being will reach optimum health and total efficiency given the ideal conditions that each is genetically designed to achieve. I believe with all my heart and soul that we are genetically designed to eat a species-specific diet of fresh, ripe organic fruits. It's that simple and pure. On this basis, I will introduce my favorite fruit.

Avocados

This fruit is my go-to food for calories and fat. Avocados are one of those nonassuming fruits that really don't stand out as a yummy-to-the-tummy fruit. Its green color, in most cases, is a real turnoff to a lot of people.

Most avocados are small and able to fit snuggly in your palm. The reason I like them is because their fat content is about 75 percent. For whatever reason, I absolutely crave them about 11 a.m. It's like a sparkling diamond whose richness, blandness, smooth texture and creamy softness becomes my nirvana of happiness. Eating an avocado totally satiates me giving me a feeling of fullness. I generally eat one to one-and-a-half avocados a day.

Avocados are so easy to eat. I pick up one up, split it in half with knife and then eat it, straight up. No preparation is required. This way of eating is great for anyone who has little time to prepare, cook and clean up after meals. The fact of the matter is that with this way of eating, there isn't any food waste—only scraps and peels, which can be composted. I began composting in 2011 and love it! There's no plastic, recyclables and trash. What else can you ask for?

Bananas

Bananas are my rock, keeping me charged, fit and young. They are a calorie- and nutrient-dense food, averaging about 100 calories each. They are probably one of my four key dietary choices on a daily basis. I begin my day by eating six to eight bananas in the morning as my breakfast between 10 a.m. and noon. Keep in mind the "love" part. Bananas are simple to eat, supertasty and require less than an hour to digest completely. That, my friends, is pure love. You are giving the body one fruit at a time, meaning the body has only one conversation at a time. This means the body can use its total life force to uptake, transport and deliver these vital nutrients to where the body needs it in a matter of minutes, not days.

Green Smoothies

In my ideal world, my first taste of food is at 10 a.m., eating about five or six bananas followed by a green smoothie loaded with five to seven bananas plus pears, apples, leafy green vegetables and water. This smoothie lasts me two days. Combined with my breakfast of bananas and lunch, which includes an avocado, my calorie count comes to 1,400 for the day. My day is set.

Tomatoes

Tomatoes are also are my go-to food. For whatever reason, I am attracted like clockwork to eating them between noon and 4 p.m. With its shiny red color, the tomato is the kind of fruit I can eat with no thought as to preparation. It's my natural instinct to tune inward and say, "Arnold, eat them now." So I do.

I generally eat tomatoes whole. I just grab them and eat— it's no big deal. They are easy to grab and eat. As with avocados and bananas, tomatoes are tasty, attractive to the eye and, more important, are made from love. When we eat these fruits in this way, we are giving love to ourselves. It's a perfect match.

Leafy Greens

Romaine lettuce and other leafy greens, as labeled by Victoria Boutenko, *Green for Life* author, is a distinct class from the vegetable family and is the other key component to a super healthy lifestyle.[5] I'll discuss more about Victoria's work in Chapter 16. I shoot to eat a pound of leafy greens a day. This can be done very easily by adding a whole head of romaine lettuce, which is about 100 calories, to a green smoothie. According to David Klein and his research for his book *Your Natural Diet: Alive Raw Foods*, greens are loaded with minerals. He suggests that 4 percent of our daily calorie requirements should be based on leafy greens.

I eat other leafy greens such as spinach, red leaf lettuce and spring mix. I am not a big fan of kale or collard greens, but these leafy vegetables are high in minerals and taste really great in green smoothies.

Celery

Celery is one of my favorite vegetables. I ideally try to eat, blend or juice celery daily. I like to eat it by itself. I just get a few celery sticks and graze on them throughout the day. There was a short period of several weeks in which I became obsessed with celery and dates combined. I began eating 10 to 15 dates with celery. This did wonders for my bowel movements, which went from two to three a day to four to five, sometimes six. I was in heaven, thinking all the plaque, all the buildup over the years is finally being removed! Unfortunately, I noticed my teeth were beginning to turn brown so I stopped—and everything returned to normal.

I now make sure I add dates to my green smoothies and eat dates in very small quantities. I eat celery by itself primarily because it tastes good, and no preparation time is required.

Dates

Dates are one of the foods I eat daily no matter what. Dates are the "magical mystery tour" of life's essential requirements. They keep me buzzed and provide me with a zest for enjoying each moment of my life. It's one of those fruits that sneak up on you, taps you on the shoulder and brings you across the finish line, so to speak. Dates are a major source of my calories.

Dates and bananas are calorie- and nutrient-rich foods, which I thrive on. A date comprises about 55 calories. My day, including morning exercise, runs from about 6 a.m. to 10:30 p.m., which is 16-and-a-half hours, with very little down time. I need 2,500 to 3,000 calories a day. I also am very physically active in my store, picking up boxes, stocking shelves, preparing food for patrons and cleaning up. Between eating avocados, bananas, tomatoes and dates, I eat almost 2,000 calories. My daily calorie requirement is pretty much set, so I don't have to worry about binging or craving. When I don't eat enough during a day, however, I get cravings.

Watermelon

During the summer, when watermelon is widely available, I pretty much forget about most other fruits. I eat an average of a half to a whole watermelon a day. Its 92 percent water composition makes it act as a supercleanser for all parts of the body. Additionally, eating watermelon requires almost no energy for digestion.

Besides being tasty and delicious to eat, that watermelon is 92 percent water means eating it is almost like going on a water fast. This means very little energy is needed for digestion, giving the body more time to go to areas of the body that need repair or waste removal. I am not a believer in colonics for this reason. I believe the body has its own built-in intelligence to do the job once the digestive energy is reduced.

Watermelon is a key food that enables one to cleanse and continue working or going about day-to-day activities. In my opinion, it is more effective than juicing, which is labor-intensive and not as cost-effective. A rule of thumb for juicing is to drink only eight to 10 ounces per hour. I did this kind of juice fast for 30 days and also ate only watermelon for 35 days. I am well-aware of the requirements and results of these fasts. Knowing what I know now, I would not do these kinds of fasts again unless in a controlled environment where I could focus completely on resting. In both cases, I worked the entire time. All this said, even though juicing and eating watermelon were not done in ideal conditions, both fasts were highly beneficial for me.

Knowing what I know today, if you want to get super-charged, supercleansed and superclear, I strongly suggest eating just watermelon for no more than 10 days or so rather than juicing.

Cherries and Grapes

Cherries and grapes are summertime foods to me. I love them—they are like a vacation food in my mouth. Being a simple guy, my needs are extremely minimal. I feel honored and blessed just by seeing and tasting these marvelous little fruits using this thought process as a basis.

Blackberries

To me, blackberries are a work of art. It feels like an artist used all his or her skills to create these multifaceted berries. I feel so honored eating them. To me, they are a super treat.

Mangoes

I have to be in the mood to eat mangoes. I like them but don't love them. I do like the way they have to be eaten. I generally quarter them and then peel the skin off. My friend, Megan, swears by them. They are her main calorie source.

She averages eight to 10 a day. Each mango is between 130-150 calories.

Durian

I can't leave out durian. It smells really bad—like onion and garlic mixed—with sulfur as a byproduct, giving off a horrendous odor to the average person. To me, it's a knowing scent that says love is in the air and a durian is nearby. The actual fruit, which I generally buy frozen, is of the consistency of creamy custard with a banana filling and an éclair cream. Durian is the fruitarian package of all the yummy, totally decadent foods I loved as a kid. I love it. It's high in fat and calories, but I like to have it as a once-in-awhile treat.

The gist of why I eat the way I eat is based on love, and I think food is meant to be fuel, not entertainment. In my way of thinking, what works best for my body is eating one fruit at a time like I love one person at a time.

I can go on and on about the fruits I eat individually as a grazing meal. I always shoot for choosing fruits labeled as organic because in the back of my mind, I envision pesticides being put on fruits that are not labeled organic—yuck. However, I will still eat nonorganic fruits when organic fruits are unavailable. Keep in mind that we are not living in an ideal world. I do the best I can daily given the circumstances in which I find myself.

Chapter 16

The Green Smoothie

THE BEST WAY TO EAT is for rejuvenation, calories and ease of time. My go-to food almost daily is the green smoothie. I have been teaching classes for about 13 years. In this time, I have stressed we should eat fruits as our main source of calories and fuel. In my highest estimation, of all the thousands of people I've lectured, I figure no more than 10 people—and that number is high—have stuck to the program. It's not natural in an unnatural setting. Most people cannot sit down day after day and week after week and eat just fruits for breakfast, lunch and dinner. Most of the time, I eat in this way, but I do eat cooked food two or three times a week. I generally eat potatoes or other cooked vegetables, rice or beans with salads or an avocado. These are not the best choices in an ideal world, but they're not the worst.

Victoria Boutenko wrote a book called *Green for Life* in which she writes about the benefits of drinking green smoothies daily. In my experience, green smoothies are the salvation for not only Americans but the world. I began introducing the benefits of green smoothies in my classes about five years ago and, since doing so, a sizeable percentage of my customers drink them regularly—some even daily—helping them consume more fruits and veggies. I am not sure why, but green smoothies succeed at doing this. The percentage of people staying raw or, at the very least, incorporating more fruit and veggies into their daily diets, has increased dramatically at my store. Best yet, the people who drink green smoothies daily are enjoying tremendous results.

Life is a journey. We shoot for the ideal, but we must also realize that what is most essential is that we listen to and honor what works. My friends, for whatever reason, green smoothies work. They have changed my life, business and classes completely! I am forever indebted to Victoria Boutenko for spreading the word about green smoothies.

I was introduced to green smoothies by an email I received from Victoria Boutenko. At the time, my beard was turning white. At the time, I believed something in my diet was amiss. I was eating mostly fruits, nuts and seeds with a small amount of cooked foods thrown into the mix.

My personality is intense, obsessive and relentless to the point where, once I get a hold of a new idea, thought or question that resonates with me, it takes over my whole sense of being and I am driven to find a solution. I needed to know why my beard was turning white. It took me almost six months to discover the reason. My prior understanding was based on two key factors, but I could not fully embrace them at the time.

I recalled reading and seeing photos of Ann Wigmore, who, at the age of 50, had completely white hair. When I saw a picture of what she looked like at 80, her hair was totally black. In her case, the magic pill was wheatgrass and sprouts, with lots of juicing. For me, it was somewhat difficult to align my thought process with this approach because I wasn't a big believer in these methods. One can't argue with results, however.

I wanted my beard back to being all black but wasn't quite sure whether I was prepared to eat sprouts and drink wheatgrass juice. The very thought of consuming them, in the back of my mind, was unnatural. What is a man to do? I had to live my highest truth, which is that fruit is the key factor in achieving the highest health possible, and let Wigmore's theory and results linger in my thought process.

At the time, I also thought about monkeys and, specifically, bonobos because everything I read at the time indicated their DNA structure is very similar in design to humans'. I was 99.4 percent sure the solution to my dilemma was connected in some way to what I was reading about bonobos, but there was still something I missed. I kept asking myself why my beard was turning gray. My fascination with bonobos and concern about my graying beard weighed heavily on me. I needed to know—I needed an answer. It was just a matter of time before I figured it out.

Then one magical day, like getting hit by a bolt of lightning or seeing fireworks on the Fourth of July, I knew what I had to do. Everything I sought on my quest came to an abrupt end. I found the solution, and it resonated with every part of my soul and the very core of my being. I received an email from Victoria Boutenko telling me about *Green for Life*, her new book at the time. In this book, she writes about her research, desire for truth and synopsis on how the body should operate given ideal foods.[5] Her quest was my quest. Whereas I thought and thought, she researched and researched. Given this synchronicity in thought process, even though we were 3,000 miles apart and really don't communicate despite my knowing her personally and having only the highest regard for her and her work, it was a magical moment of divine communication. When I began reading her email, I was intrigued and impressed—and began to realize my life was about to take a dramatic leap to the next level, wherever it would be.

In *Green for Life*, Victoria explains her research and, more important, the results of that research. She writes about Wigmore's failing health and how she began to revitalize herself once she began adding wheatgrass, sprouts and juicing to her dietary regimen.5 In conclusion, her daily dietary consumption also completely changed by giving up all processed foods.5 This lighted up all kinds of cautionary green lights in me and made me consider that perhaps her research could be my salvation in discovering what was amiss in my diet, causing my beard to go white.

In this book, Victoria explains how we, as a species, are most closely related to bonobos based on DNA structure.5 She discusses what and how bonobos eat.5 She writes about how they are eaters of mostly fruits with greens mixed in.5 At that time, I could not believe that someone who was 3,000 miles away, who I never spoke or wrote to, could come to the same conclusions with the exact same identification guidelines as Wigmore about bonobos.

The next paragraph I read was the clincher for me. The next paragraph not only turned my life around but led to a dramatic increase in my business within a day at my store. Victoria writes about her husband's beard as being gray at the time and says once he began drinking large quantities of green smoothies, his gray beard turned black.5 When I read that sentence, all these stars and lights went off in my brain. It was like: *Presto!* and *bingo!* I had found my answer as to what I needed to do for my beard to go back to black. I had my answer as to what was missing in my diet. I had my answer as to what has to be shared over and over as the key ingredient for what it takes to be raw, live raw and stay raw.

So on that note, I thank Victoria Boutenko for her driving force of truth. I appreciate her sharing what works and what doesn't work. After reading this information in *Green for Life*, I completely changed the focus of my business. I went from promoting an organic raw vegan lifestyle with a focus on banana whips, a raw vegan version of ice cream using frozen fruits, to a focus on green smoothies as being the key recipe to becoming vibrantly healthy.

As it was then as it is now, in my opinion, eating whole fruits and leafy greens daily is the ideal way to eat. This being said, in my experience, of all the thousands of people I've taught, less than a handful can stay on this lifestyle approach day after day, month after month and year after year, as I noted earlier. In our society, we are bombarded by mass media programming that dictates our dietary choices. These media outlets hammer at us from the moment we wake up that we should smell the fresh aroma of coffee, buy donuts and eat a hearty breakfast of eggs, bacon and home fries. We listen to the radio, watch TV commercials, go to school and out to eat, drive our cars, walk down streets and take a trip down memory lane to our childhoods, where we have memories of being rewarded as a kid with treats. We, as a people, are doomed—for lack of a better word—to continue in the dietary framework that has been established.

In my experience, the green smoothie is the white knight or bolt of greased lightning that will be the driving force that will empower one to unshackle all those negative, built-in mass media influences on dietary products.

In my experience, once one begins drinking a minimum of 32 ounces of green smoothies every day for a month, one undergoes a change of consciousness and begins to take responsibility for his or her health. The reason for this is that green smoothies are loaded with fruits, the basic fuel for every cell in our bodies. Fruit is the primary gas that keeps our bodies running. Without this major source of power, the body begins break down and degenerate. The body can still operate but requires more work to convert other foods into a useable power source. Fruits and veggies (greens) provide the highest forms of vitamins, minerals, essential fatty acids and other nutrients that is most usable by our bodies.

The secret as to why green smoothies are such a powerful nutrient sources is that all the fruits and leafy greens are blended into a predigested state, requiring little time for the body to break down. On a day-to-day basis, the body's goal is purification and homeostasis. If the body spends little energy on digestion, its remaining energy capacity will go to detoxification and rejuvenation and whatever is required by the body for optimum health. As the body is given more energy to systematically cleanse and purify the body, it will become clear about what is the best dietary choice for optimum health and well-being.

My friends, green smoothies represent the key to achieving the highest nutrient source for the body, from what I have seen. Without green smoothies, it is very hard to maintain being raw. Remember, food is meant not to entertain but to fuel the body. Green smoothies are easy to make and nutrient-dense, with very little time required for digestion. Enough said. By the way, I drink at least 32 ounces of green smoothie a day. My beard did not completely turn to black, but at the very least, it is not getting white anymore. At the most, my beard is getting darker. So I give my highest thanks to Victoria.

Chapter 17

The 5–5–5 Rule

I ADVOCATE SOMETHING called the 5–5–5 Rule:

- **A meal should have no more than 5 ingredients.**
- **A meal should cost no more than $5.**
- **A meal should take no more than 5 minutes to prepare.**

What the heck does this mean? It means most raw foods recipes are too fancy, containing too many ingredients and too much oil, in the form of nuts and spices. They are complicated, hard to make and take too long to prepare. They should be made only on special occasions and for bragging rights. If one is to be serious about raw foods, he or she has to indulge in a lifestyle that is most conducive to optimum health. One has to eat according to his or her body's ultimate needs. Our bodies need to be treated with love by eating in the way I've described for optimum health. The 5–5–5 rule is the way to get more clarity and feel superhealthy with a more positive outlook. This will enhance one's ability to feel better emotionally and gain excellent health and overall well-being.

The primary rule for making a superhealthy dish is:

A meal should have no more than 5 ingredients.

This is basically self-explanatory. If a meal contains more than 5 ingredients, the food will take longer to digest and process and longer for the body to assimilate the food. It will also take longer to deliver and transport all the vital nutrients to wherever they should go.

Ingredients have to meet three basic requirements before they are eaten:

- **Was the food grown in nature?** This means that anything that nature provides can be eaten provided it meets the other 2 requirements.

- **Was the food found on a tree, bush or vine or the ground**? Once again, nature is, by design, for our benefit. It does not need to be improved upon. It is perfect in its natural form, having the energy of the sun, moon and earth and the water, all of which contain the universal power of life, which has taken millions of years to perfect.

- **Is the food yummy to the tummy?** This is a key element to this lifestyle. This is what separates the men from the boys, what separates truth from lies, what is good for our bodies to eat and what is not. There is no gray area, and there is no, "I guess" and no questions as to whether it's good or bad for our bodies. If one cannot eat anything in large quantity that is raw, ripe and fresh from the garden, it means we are not genetically designed to eat it. This means that all oils, which are 100 percent fat, all salts, which can gag, if not kill, you almost instantaneously even if eaten in small quantities, let alone in large quantities, should never be eaten. Garlic, which causes our mouths to spit up like a bad dream, should never be eaten. The same goes for all condiments such as pepper, ginger or any spice, which supposedly enhances the flavor of food but sets up our bodies to go on full-scale military alerts to neutralize and eliminate the condiments'.

These are the rules of life. There is no middle ground, no gray areas. Our bodies thrive on being in a state of perfection and harmony. Any food or recipe ingredient we put into our mouths has to meet these requirements so it can be enjoyed. Keep in mind that I am talking about following this practice in an ideal world. Keep in mind that wherever you are in the big scheme of things, enjoy your life. Keep in mind that self love ranks the highest order. Food represents a part of the whole picture. It's a big part, but not the whole picture.

In my mind, breakfast and dinner are the most important meals, which must meet these requirements ideally. Initially, lunch can be a cheat meal, but I recommend that a salad precede these cheat meals. In the long term, you will lose the desire for cheat meals but you'll find the body demands excellence in diet at all times. If you stray toward cooked and complicated fare, enjoy it and then get back on track the next day so your body can catch up.

A meal should cost no more than $5.

This means that fruit is cheap once you understand fruits will be your main source of fuel. In the United States, farmers' markets; Community Supported Agriculture, or CSAs; and wholesale distributors are available, and you can't beat the prices. Even if you bought conventionally grown bananas, seven bananas at 700 calories represents the ultimate fast food. These bananas can be bought at almost any convenience store, grocery store or supermarket, costing less than $1 sometimes. I challenge any fast-food chain to come up with something that compares with bananas in cost and nutrient value. Already, it is beyond impossible and totally inconceivable for fast-food restaurants to prepare and package a food in the amount of time it takes to peel a banana.

A meal should take no more than 5 minutes to prepare.

Eating whole fruits using just your hands, the best tools out there, means no preparation time. Blending is the next easiest route to take. Just put a whole bunch of fruit in a blender and, within two minutes, your meal is ready. Raw foods should be simple, cost-effective and time-manageable, which is perfect for everyone. It is the perfect food!

Chapter 18

My Daily Food Choices

IN MY OPINION, as explained earlier, my high-calorie choice:

Bananas
- I eat 10 to 15 a day.
- I put five to seven bananas in my green smoothie.
- I eat three to five bananas straight up.
- I eat five bananas in a banana whip. I'll generally add dates and carob to the whip.

Dates
- I eat five to 10 per day. Each date is about 55 calories.

Avocados
- I also eat one-and-a-half avocados, which are high in fat but easily digestible.

These are my high-calorie foods. I pick and graze the rest. Dinner is either fruit or spaghetti, which is spiralized zucchini with tomato, red pepper, mangoes and dates, pulsed in a food processor, about five times and served over spaghetti.

And that, my friends, is the majority of my food day. The secret is that I do this day in and day out, month in and month out, year in and year out. It is my opinion, based on what I know, experience and envision, that if we follow this lifestyle to at least 50 percent raw vegan, not only will the disease rate be greatly reduced but the crime rate will plummet. Warring between people and nations would be greatly reduced, and our environment would stop being destroyed by harmful thoughts and creations so prevalent to make money.

Hence, my lifetime purpose and mission, "To create an energetic movement for the transformation of a disease free world," will become a reality.

It is my opinion, in each and every one of us, there exists a godly way of being that brings not only peace and harmony in us but gives us the power to create peace out in the world.

Chapter 19

Dry Fasting

I LOVE *QUANTUM EATING* by Tonya Zavastas and her—even though we've never met. Her book appears to me to come from more of a research-based scientific level, intertwined with her experience.

When I talk about *Quantum Eating* to customers, I generally refer to a section in which she talks about water and the idea of dry fasting.[6] She tells us that not only can we stop the aging process by performing a dry fast but can reverse the aging process and stay young.[6] I love it. I don't want to age and, in my belief, haven't aged much in the 14 years since I began a raw vegan lifestyle.

Tanya is a strong proponent of dry fasting for 15 hours a day as well as getting your total water source from only fruits and veggies.[6] At this particular time in my life, I agree with Tanya's stance on this topic and try to follow her advice daily.

Water is a controversial subject among everyone, including raw foodists. The bottom-line is that your body knows best. Listen to no one as the final say. If this advice resonates with you, however, follow it for a while. In my case, the idea of taking in no water and dry fasting for 15 hours from 7 p.m. to 10 a.m. resonated with my inner innate intelligence, which told me this protocol was the perfect method to enhance my body's optimum health performance.

Chapter 20

Favorite Books

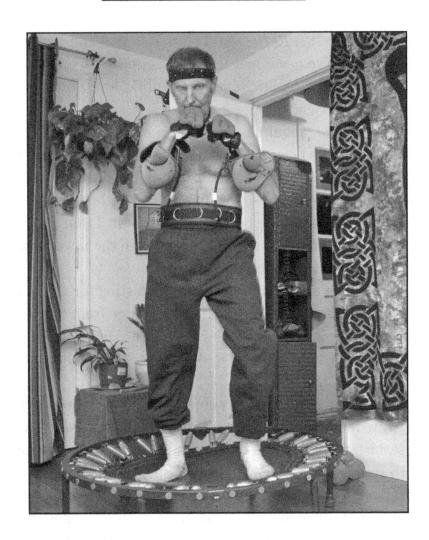

THE FINAL CHAPTER reinforces what I believe and serves as a way to share it with others. For whatever reason, people come to my store to seek answers as to why they have a certain disease, and they ask, "Why me?" It is my job to share my truth on whichever disease or condition they have and to let them know the affliction can be greatly improved by going raw. I not only want to share with my patrons, shedding some light on the subject of their suffering, but provide answers that can help them. It is on this basis that I choose the following books.

I answer the questions they have as best I can. But who am I? I'm not a doctor, nutritionist or someone who has done any medical research to discover the in-depth cause of any diseases or conditions. I am just a simple man who is passionate about what he does and shares information with anyone who wants to hear what I have to say.

As I share, I refer. As I give out flyers, I show pages from a continual flow of books. I do whatever it takes for my customers to believe in themselves, their innate healing system and the idea that in taking responsibility for their health, they can get closer to their goal of improving their diseases or conditions. I tell them that, in the end, they are the only ones they can depend upon. On this basis, I would like to share some of my favorite books, which had a tremendous influence not only on me but my customers.

1. *The 80/10/10 Diet* by Doug Graham

This is the most provocative book of our time. It's a detailed, compelling book that is easily comprehended by the masses. It draws on the fact that raw is not only doable but necessary for humans to maintain optimum health. It's a step-by-step approach on why we should eat a mostly fruitarian diet based on the laws of nature. It is the most-sold book and my go-to book that deals with research on a raw foods diet. It is the one book that doctors do not want you to read. It is the one book that can help one constructively change their dietary habits.

2. *Raw Family* by Victoria, Igor, Sergei and Valya Boutenko

This book has probably influenced more people to go raw or, at the very least, to think seriously about going raw than any other book I know. It's a story about a family who, against all odds and all conventional thinking, and facing serious health challenges, healed each and every one of themselves of asthma to Type 1 diabetes just by changing to an all-raw lifestyle,

I highly recommend this extremely inspiring book. It's easy reading about an unforgettable family whose journey from eating the standard American diet to leading an all-raw food lifestyle produced amazing results. Still to this day, this life-changing book has made a worldwide impact on our daily dietary choices.

3. *Green for Life* by Victoria Boutenko

This is one of those nonassuming books that no one would ever think its material would have such worldwide impact. But this book and its implication though research and actual testing has literally and figuratively had such a dramatic influence on all aspects of my life, all my customers' lives and thousands of others. See Chapter 16 on green smoothies. It is in this regard that I am forever indebted to Victoria for her willingness to share her research and applications of these findings with all of us.

Look at the chapters on green smoothies, hypothyroid, Vitamin B12, chronic fatigue and candida.

This book is a great testimonial on why green smoothies work to vastly improve one's health. I can't say enough about it. I highly recommend this book.

4. Self Healing Colitis & Crohn's by David Klein

There are very few books I have any desire to read once, let alone twice. This book, however, is like I found gold. It has so much in-depth information that is easy to read and understand. I can read this book over and over and still not get tired of it.

There is so much pertinent information on so many different pages on how to obtain optimum health that it takes two or three readings to comprehend the full gist of all the information David provides.

I personally refer to his chapter on inflammation almost daily. This chapter deals with aches and pains and how it is one's benefit to have it. This concept is so foreign to the average American that, upon reading it for the first time, he or she will have all these "a-ha" moments about the body's intelligence and its ongoing pursuit of perfection. Every questionable theory out there is explained away. This book is a must-read.

This is one of the best comprehensive books I have ever read. In my opinion, it's not necessary to buy a lot of books. Choose the authors who resonate with you the most and read their books over and over.

Self Healing Colitis & Crohn's is one of those timeless books that has to be read over and over till one gets it. I take my hat off (if I had a hat) to David Klein for his words, his experience and his willingness to share his truth.

5. *The Live Food Factor* by Susan Schenck

This book is huge. It has more 600 pages and is filled with so much information that I had to take breaks just to absorb everything. This book should be the bible for those who want an in-depth report on why to go raw with an emphasis on fruit. This book, as quoted on front cover, is "the comprehensive guide to the ultimate diet for body, mind, spirit and planet," and it is just that. What I really love about this book is that for each topic, it gives many sides with no absolute answer and allows the reader to ultimately decide which path is the best to take.

The Live Food Factor contains so many good points. It's more than any memory can handle. Whenever a new customer walks into my store, I generally tell him or her that *Live Food Factor* has an answer. In other words, it's a very comprehensive volume about why leading a raw vegan lifestyle is recommended and the dramatic effect it has on one during the change to this lifestyle.

6. *Raw Food Treatment of Cancer* by Kristine Nolfi

This is my go-to book if I have a consultation with any woman regarding any health issue. This book demands attention. It's about an M.D. living in Denmark who went against conventional medical treatment when diagnosed with a tumor the size of a hen's egg growing in her breast. It is the story of a doctor who realized that raw food is the key factor in the treatment of cancer. When she began treating her patients with raw foods, her colleagues noticed not her success with those patients who were so far gone and yet completely healed by leading a raw foods lifestyle but the fact that, under her care, two patients died. She was forced to give up her medical practice.

7. *The Miracle of Fasting* by Paul C. and Patricia Bragg

I read this book about 10 years ago, and it made such an impression on me that I adopted a lot of the Braggs' suggestions in my lifestyle. For example, Paul wrote: "Earn you breakfast fasting for 12-15 hours daily. Get exercise and sunshine." He had a strong belief in the body's healing ability. The book is based on fasting and how it is the body's innate healing system—the ultimate healer. Paul Bragg lived, practiced, taught and experienced through working with thousands of people that fasting from all food except for water was very healing to the body. He tells us that when the body is freed from the digestive process, it prioritizes which internal organs and tissues are the most polluted and doing the most harm. It will then begin the cleansing process. There are 250 pages of fact-filled information that I read at least three times and reference countless times.

Paul's body was amazing. This was a man who lived his principles. What he did physically at age 80 is almost impossible by someone in their 20s. His secret was fasting.

I have fasted seven times from three to 21 days and no longer have any desire to fast regularly. It's not that I don't believe fasting is beneficial and cleansing and can be of extreme benefit to anyone who does it for a minimum of three days. The reason I feel this way is that the body, for the first three days, is focused on using the sugar in the body as fuel. It is not until the fourth day that the body goes to the adipose tissue, which contains much acid residue, and converts it to usable fuel or figures out a way to dispose of it.

With that said and considering the benefits derived from that procedure, I prefer dry fasting on a daily basis for 12 to 15 hours. According to Tonya Zavastas' *Quantum Eating*, dry fasting is shown to be just as, if not more, effective than water fasting. Nevertheless, my feelings are mixed on this matter. If I ran into a serious mold allergic reaction or had a bug bite, I would resort to a more-intensive cleansing procedure with water fasting if dry fasting for one or two days wasn't sufficient.

8. *The Raw Life* by Paul Nison

This is my go-to book for any meat eater who walks in to my store. Paul explains what meat does to your body and breaks it down to a simple, easy-to-read format.

Paul's incisive commentary regarding meat consumption makes me dazzle. I liken this challenge to sparring with a boxing opponent. I love it so. I jab and I punch away at this core belief in my customers. So with each new customer who has a question on health, the Raw Life is my go-to book. He lists page after page on how meat items are produced and processed and what they do to your body.

I have known Paul about 15 years. We got involved with raw foods almost at the same time. *The Raw Life* was his first book. I liked it back then and I still like it today.

9. *Avoiding Degenerative Disease* by Don Bennett

I carry about 150 raw foods books that cover many different ideas, recipes and thought processes. I have read most of them and know a few of the authors on a first-name basis. That said, I can say hands down that this book and this author is the most underrated in the field. On the flip side, this book will be in the top of the must-read books that anyone seeking more information on the raw foods diet has to read.

The title says it all. Everything I know and have experienced is in complete alliance with Don. I highly recommend that you read Don's book because his words and his understanding of sickness and healing through a raw vegan lifestyle resonates with me.

Don offers wonderful advice on what and what not to do. I have read this book at least twice cover to cover and use it almost every day in my practice.

10. *Food for Life* by Neal Barnard

I love this book. Although this book is not a raw foods book, Dr. Barnard totally emphasizes why not only a vegan diet is so important but why a meat-based diet is the primary cause of most disease. I refer to this book almost daily.

I love this book because it resonates with me, highlighting why eating meat is not only very unhealthy but the root cause of most diseases. Dr. Barnard explains from a medical viewpoint that what you eat will strongly determine what disease you will get. This book is a must-read.

11. *Easy To Be Raw* by Megan Elizabeth

This is the best raw vegan food-prep book I've read so far, bar none. This is the only recipe book I recommend to my customers. It's simple, easy, functional and, most important, the recipes are written in accordance with Doug Graham's 80/10/10 recommendations. Doug's program is the one I advocate the most for restoring health and rejuvenating one's body. Megan is a young woman who I personally mentored for more than three years on how to live a healthy raw vegan lifestyle. As quoted on the back jacket of *Easy to be Raw*: "Megan has changed my life forever. There's not a dish of hers I don't enjoy! I'm inspired by her integrity and I trust her completely."

Conclusion

This is it.

This is my book, my lifetime and my continuing journey into the next moment.

I was driven to write this book based on circumstances. I was driven to share my 65 years of life and how I got to where I am today. This truth is no more and no less than anyone else, but I felt I had to share my truth with all of you to help you to live a disease-free life and achieve your highest well-being and health.

This is my story to date, and I'm looking forward to the upcoming years, wherever that may take me.

I thank you.

Notes

Endnotes

[1] Diamond, Harvey and Marilyn. *Fit for Life*. New York, New York: Warner Books, 1987, 1989.

[2] Graham, Douglas N. *The 80/10/10 Diet*. Decatur, Georgia: FoodnSport Press, 2006.

[3] Walker, Norman. *Become Younger*. Summertown, Tennessee: Norwalk Press, 1949.

[4] Bennett, Don. *Avoiding Degenerative Disease*. KayLastima Publishing Company, 2006.

[5] Boutenko, Victoria. *Green for Life*. Berkeley, California: North Atlantic Books, 2005, 2010.

[6] Zavastas, Tonya. *Quantum Eating*. Cordova, Tennessee: BR Publishing, 2007.

Made in the USA
Middletown, DE
24 July 2024